AMONGST THE VILLAGE MAGAZINE

Fall 2024 Issue

Powered by the
Perinatal Resource Collaborative
A Division of HARLOT Co. &
Womb Light Energy LLC.

Founder's Welcome

Welcome to the
First Issue of the Amongst
the Village Magazine!

Within this season we are
thrilled to share resources,
stories, and information
that will educate, inspire
and empower you during
your own perinatal
journey... so that you feel
Amongst the Village.

Nicole Harlit

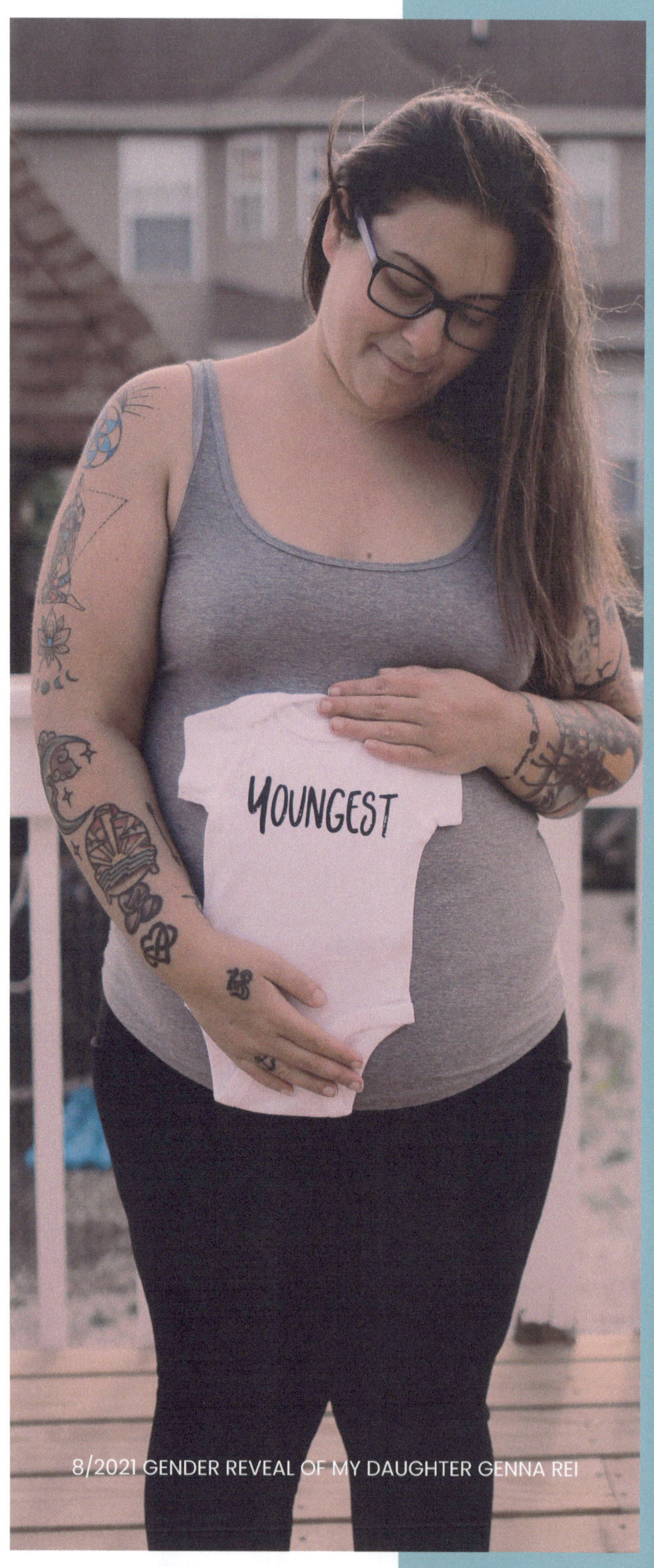

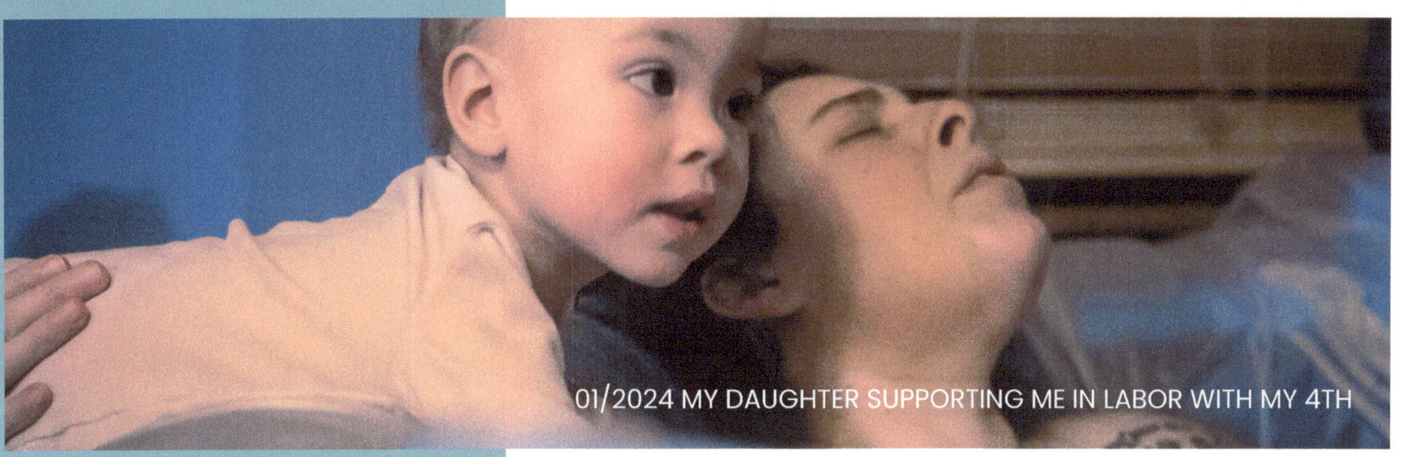

A PEEK AT WHAT'S WITHIN

Ask the Village

Submit Your Questions & See Answers from Various Members of the Village.

Founder's Spotlight

Learn a little about Nicole Harlot and her vision and mission for the magazine and beyond.

Prenatal Workouts

The benefits and resources to a strong pregnancy and postpartum.

How to Be a Consumer for Your Pregnancy

Steps to your best birth outcome start with this understanding.

How Your Partner Can Best Support You

Basic questions to prepare you for a very important conversation

Beyond the Bounce Back

Understanding more about postpartum and what you truly need to feel good and whole.

The Importance of Community

Understanding ways to be supported and mindful during the perinatal period.

The Ultimate Postpartum Healing Guide

Integrating the basics and getting to a healed physical, emotional self.

& MORE

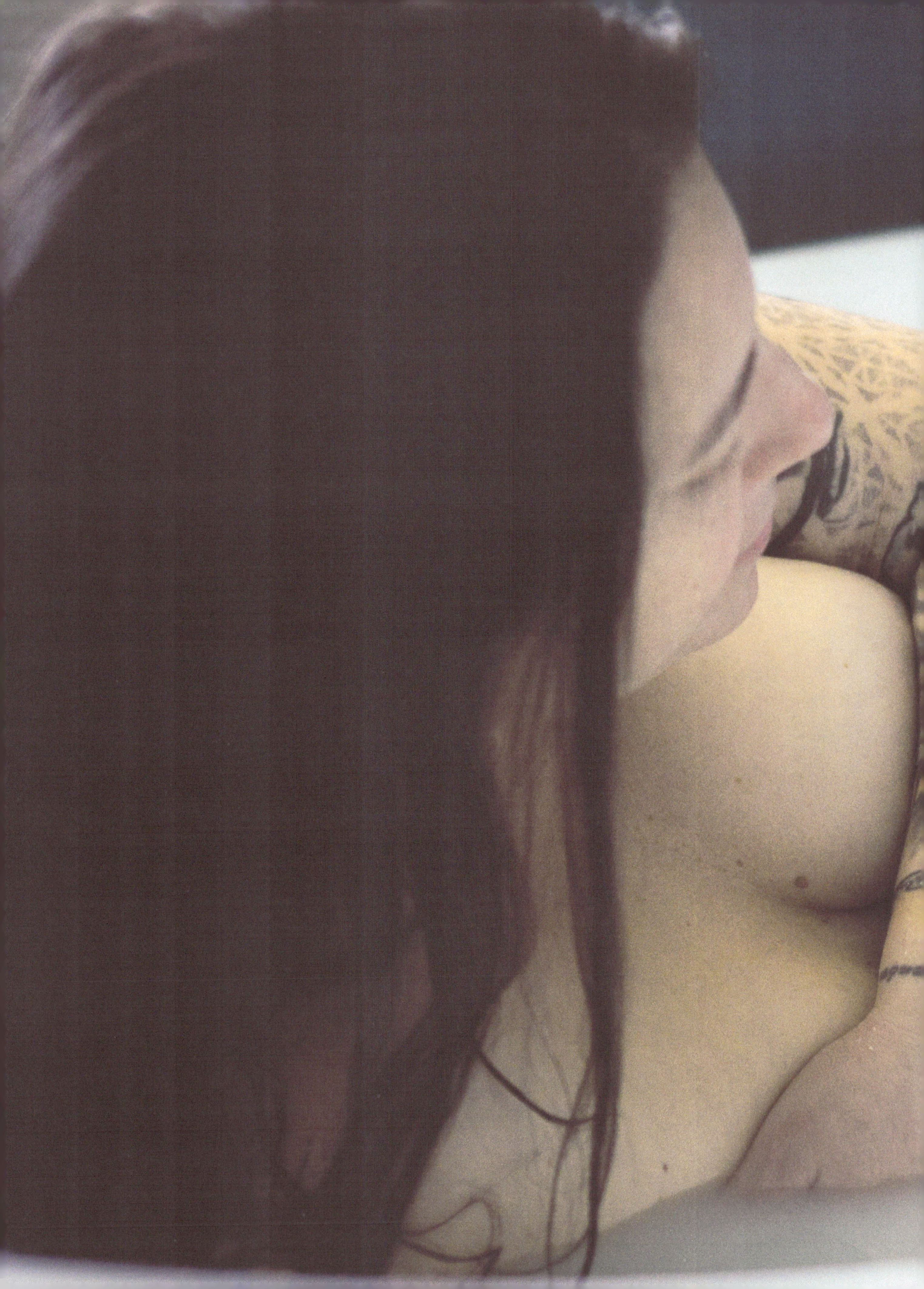

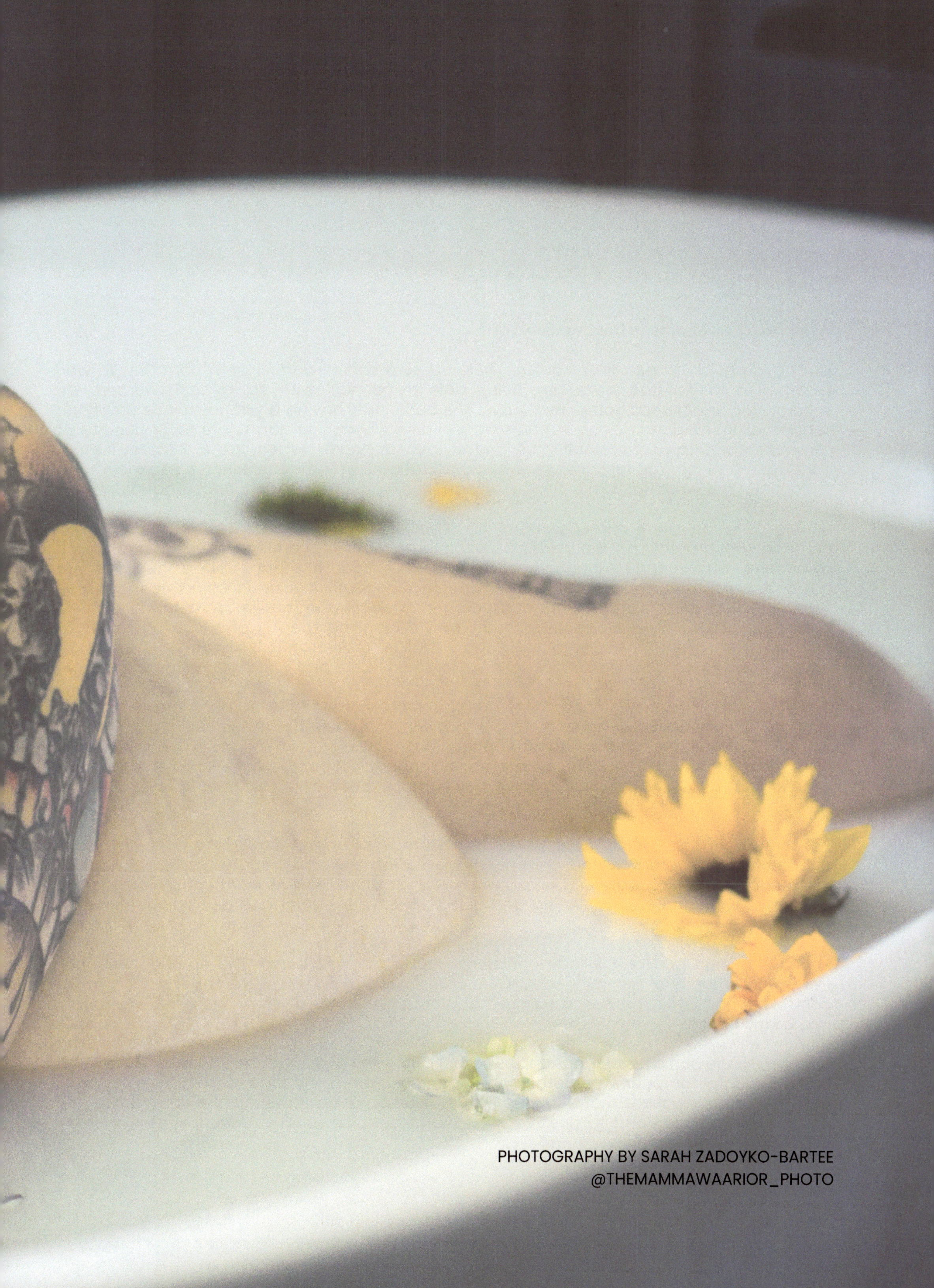

PHOTOGRAPHY BY SARAH ZADOYKO-BARTEE
@THEMAMMAWAARIOR_PHOTO

ASK THE VILLAGE

What are the benefits of having a village?

You have people to turn to for advice, help, to hold space, and most importantly, to work together in shifting the paradigm. Being able to connect with like-minded women who support and understand you is invaluable. The benefits of having a village include emotional support and self-care. Having support from others whom you can relate to or depend on allows mothers to prioritize self-care and emotional health. When you are alone, life can become too much. You feel overwhelmed, and at times, you may question if you really want to continue this work. But with a village, we can hold each other up with encouragement.

Having a village offers immense benefits, especially during significant life transitions like pregnancy and parenting. It provides essential emotional support, easing stress and anxiety by offering comfort and understanding. The collective wisdom within a village offers practical advice and solutions, making challenges more manageable. A village also provides practical help with daily tasks, reducing the burden on individuals and families. It fosters a sense of belonging, alleviating feelings of isolation, and enhancing the joy of shared experiences. Ultimately, a village empowers individuals, builds resilience, and creates a nurturing environment that makes life's challenges easier to navigate and its joys more meaningful.

Having a '*village*,' particularly an online community of women focused on prenatal care and support, offers numerous benefits. First, it provides a sense of connection and belonging, which is crucial during the prenatal period when many women may feel isolated or overwhelmed. This community serves as a supportive space where women can share experiences, ask questions, and receive advice from those who are going through or have gone through similar journeys.

Secondly, a village fosters collective wisdom. Members can tap into a wealth of knowledge and resources shared by the community, including tips on prenatal care, coping with pregnancy-related challenges, and preparing for childbirth and motherhood. This exchange of information can be empowering and help women make informed decisions about their care.

Moreover, being part of a village can boost emotional well-being. The emotional support from a community of like-minded women can reduce stress, alleviate anxiety, and provide comfort during difficult times. Knowing that others are there to listen, encourage, and uplift can be invaluable.

Lastly, a village can create opportunities for collaboration and advocacy. Together, members can advocate for better prenatal care practices, share valuable resources, and even collaborate on initiatives that benefit pregnant women and mothers in the community. This collective effort can lead to positive changes in both personal experiences and broader prenatal care standards.

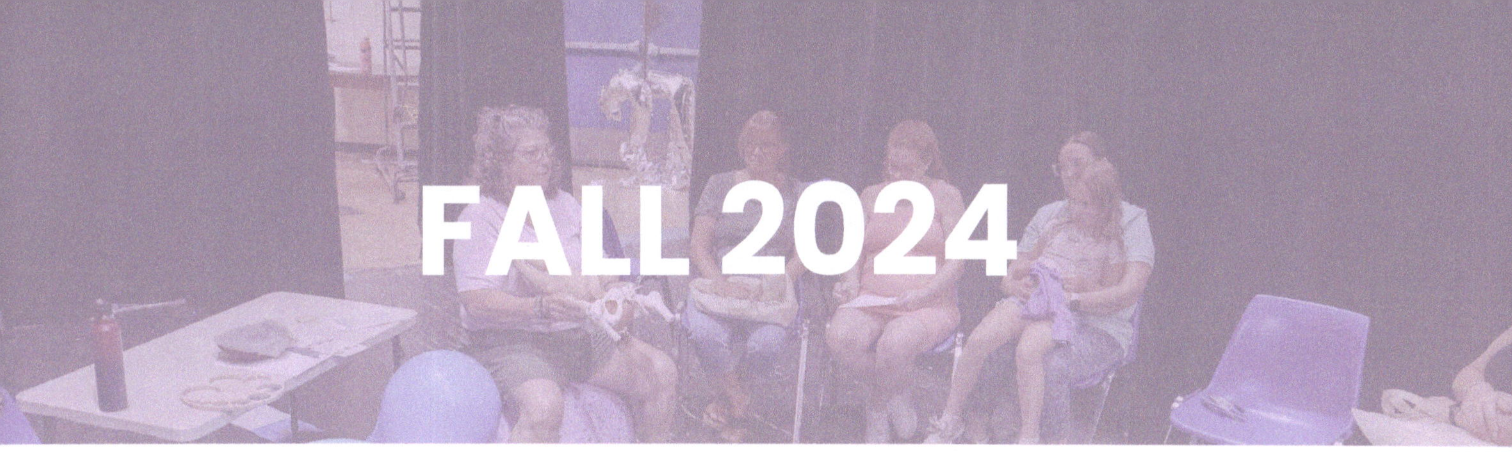

Why was having a village so important to your journey?

I have been on a healing journey ever since my first baby. Having a village has helped me get through the hard times and pulled me through them.

I need the support and motivation to do what I am wanting to do, as well as the experience of others that I can learn from. It helped me stay centered and allowed me to navigate the emotional ups and downs that come with parenthood. It allowed me to feel supported and not alone.

I would not walk across the country without a support team. I would not participate in a cancer walk without a support team. I would not go into a birth without a support team. So why would I go through life's journey without one?

My first two births ended in surgery because I was swallowed up by a system that puts financial and liability concerns above what's best for moms and babies. It wasn't until I became a doula myself and surrounded myself with other doulas, midwives, chiropractors, and so many other holistic providers that I gained the knowledge and support I needed to have the best birth and postpartum experience I could.

Loneliness can be paralyzing. We need the village to keep us strong, awake, aware, and mobilized.

Thank you to our villagers for these answers!

Melanie Sandoval, Intuitive Beginnings Doula Collective *intuitivebeginnings.info@gmail.com*
Sarah Kyle, Confident Mamas Doula LLC *confidentmamasdoula@gmail.com*
Shatiera, Seeds Of Hope LLC *shatiera@seedsofhopecc.com*
Beverly Young Reed, Full Spectrum Doula *bevdoula@gmail.com*
Dawn Thompson, Birthify, Inc. *dawn@birthify.net*
Kim Morris, Yoniversity Online Training Academy™ *trulykimmorris@gmail.com*
Christa Cornejo, A Mother's Hand Services *christa.cornejo@gmail.com*
Anne Wallen, MaternityWise International *maternitywiseinstitute@gmail.com*

Email any questions you would like answered in our next issue to prcvillage@gmail.com

Meet The Founder

By Nicole Harlot

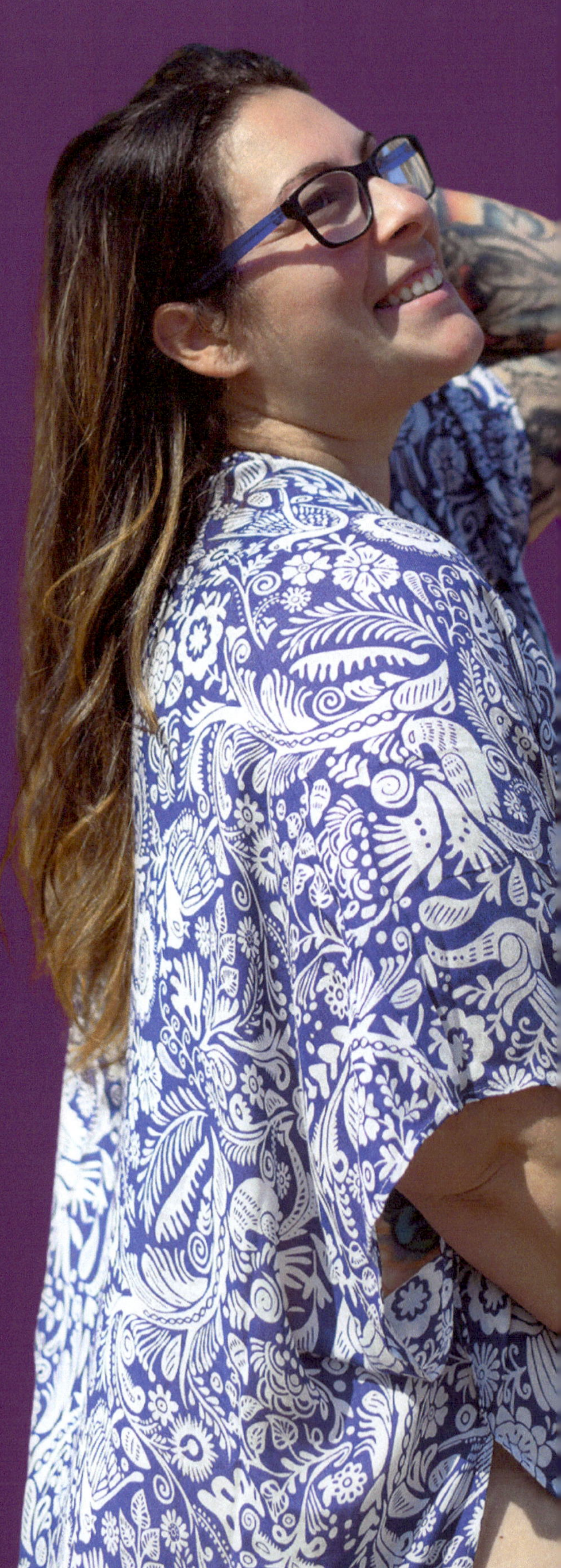

Nicole Harlot, wife and mama of four, is the Founder of the Womb Light® Energy Modality and Perinatal Alchemy. She is a Trainer and Master Practitioner of Modalities that support mind, body and energy- from NLP to Reiki. She is also an author, speaker and podcast host.

Her mission is to support women who support women and create a collective ripple of empowerment using these tools and feminine embodiment. When she isn't with her children and family or supporting others, she enjoys traveling, the beach and doing yoga.

She has trained and been mentored by some absolutely amazing women and gives her best to pay it forward to others.

Nicole has experienced an array of challenges and triumphs throughout the birth of her two boys. She went through fertility treatments and conceived her first through IUI in 2016, then survived severe PMADs after the birth of her oldest in 2017. Which launched her into the maternal support space.

In 2019, she naturally and unexpectedly conceived her second and was met with various challenges throughout her pregnancy. She went inward and listened to her body and intuition to overcome them all, and had the birth of her dreams in April 2020.

From that day, Womb Light® was also conceived and began making its way into her self healing, and ultimately to her clients.

You can find her online @perinatalalchemy
http://mag.amongstthevillage.com

Since her support network was vast from being a PMAD survivor, in August 2020, she received a download to shift her mission from directly helping womb'n to helping those who support womb'n. In September 2020, the first class of Womb Light® Practitioners was enrolled, and now there are more than 150 Practitioners worldwide. In addition, her training expanded into a full Womb Energetics & Neuro Somatics Program, which has 12 graduates in 8 beautiful modalities that support women and mothers in the perinatal period.

Now, as a mother of 4 and a perinatal professional of 7 years, she is focused on creating community for professionals and fostering collaborations to ultimately impact the collective of birthing women around the world. Her passion is cultivating the village for the villagers and creating a space where various resources, like this magazine, can be birthed and shared!

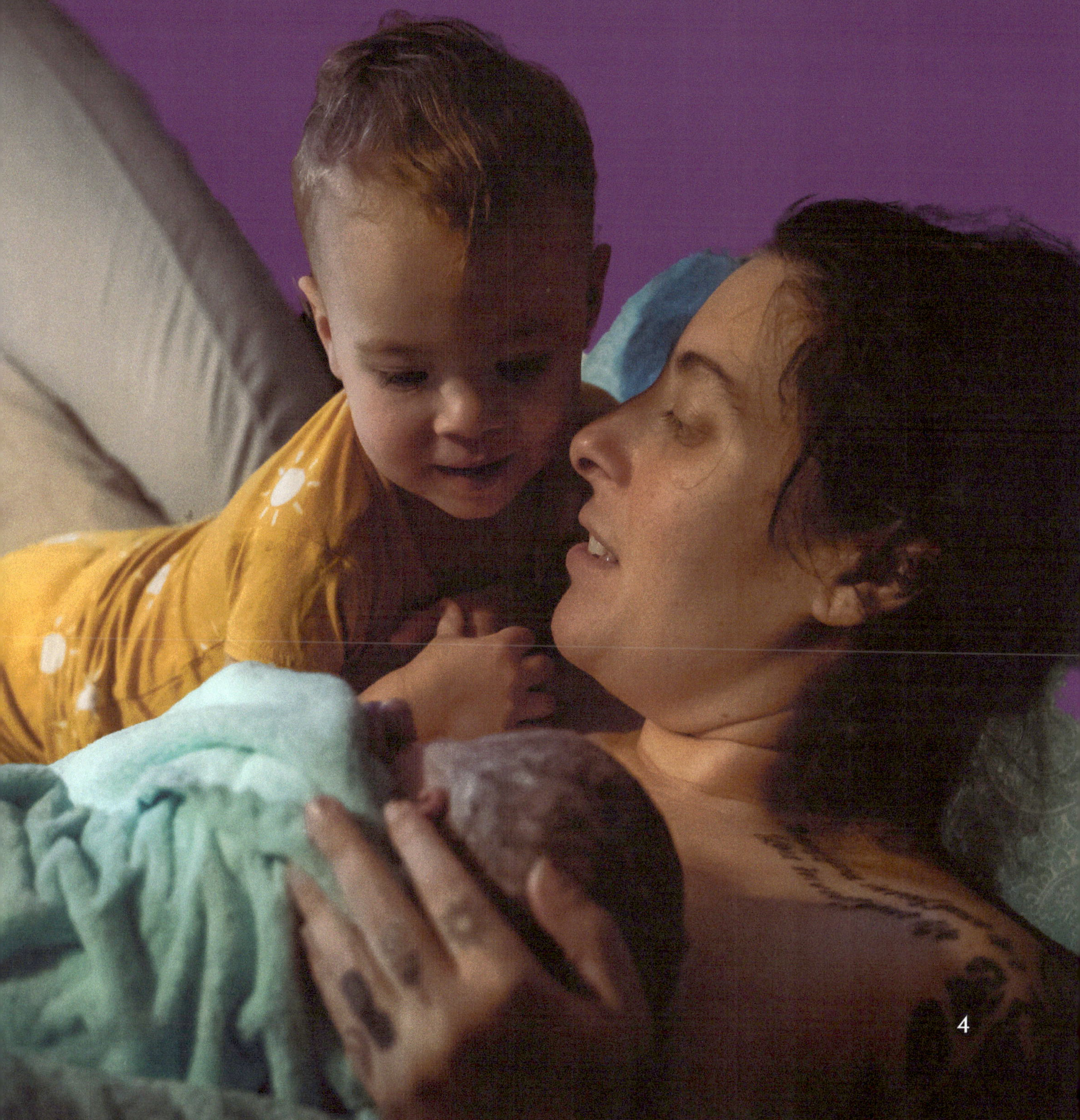

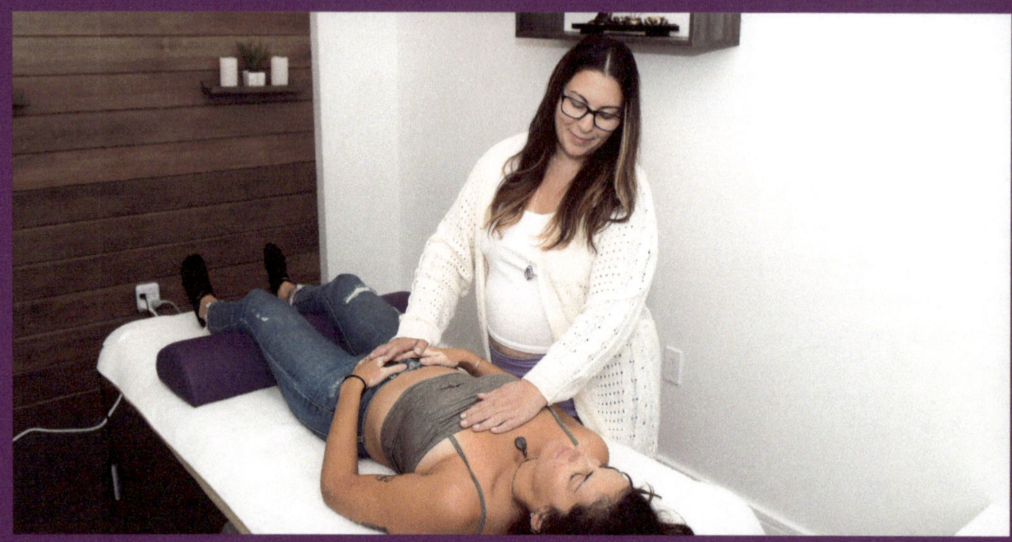

What is the Perinatal Resource Collaborative?

The Perinatal Resource Collaborative is a growing space designed to help perinatal professionals like doulas, midwives, therapists, bodyworkers, and many others thrive in all aspects of their business, cultivate relationships with others, and create resources and connections for women, mothers, and those they support.

Beyond an international virtual space, we will be building blueprints for events and opportunities within state and local communities in the future.

We invite professionals to step inside our vibrant hub, where shared resources and collective learning flourish, and multiple off-meta marketing opportunities such as a magazine and podcast are available to contribute to and share.

(Without algorithms, community standards, or sensitive content warnings getting in your way!)

The benefits and opportunities to contribute are growing and limitless. The mission is to be the village for the villagers and to fill the gaps for one another, supporting the global collective of those we serve.

If you are an expecting or new mom reading this, please share the name Perinatal Resource Collaborative with anyone who supports you during your perinatal period so they can also be supported and have opportunities to share their stories and expertise in various ways.

Together, we thrive and rise—it is a village circle.

The Village for the Villagers!
Perinatal Professionals and Providers—Join us to access all the benefits.

In this first issue, my goal is to communicate the deeper mission and the profound 'why' behind not just this magazine, but the larger vision of the Perinatal Resource Collaborative and the magic that happens when we thrive together.

Contribute to this Magazine
Be a Podcast Guest
Join Community Conversations
Networking Calls
Business Trainings
Monthly Masterclasses
Weekly Newsletter
Full Resource Library
Internal Directory Listing
External Directory Partnerships
Rewards Points Programs
Promote Your Business
Earn Commission & Bonuses

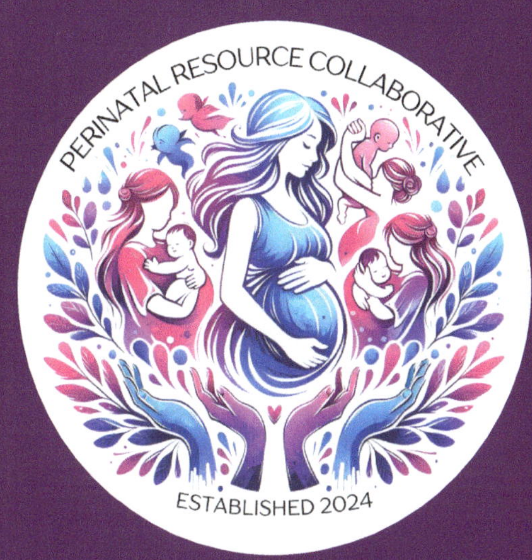

become a member today!

Nicole always reminds the community and sisterhood that she appreciates every connection made in this space. She seeks collaborative energies so that every womb'n is positively impacted and able to celebrate together.

She is fully blessed and does not take any moment of this work for granted. Please know that all Sisters, from Practitioners to Master Teachers, are such an integral part of her joy, peace, and happiness, and she is always there for you if needed!

Womb'n are truly magical creators, and she hopes that in every moment, you are reminded of that and work from that space of worthiness that comes from your Womb Light® Thank you!

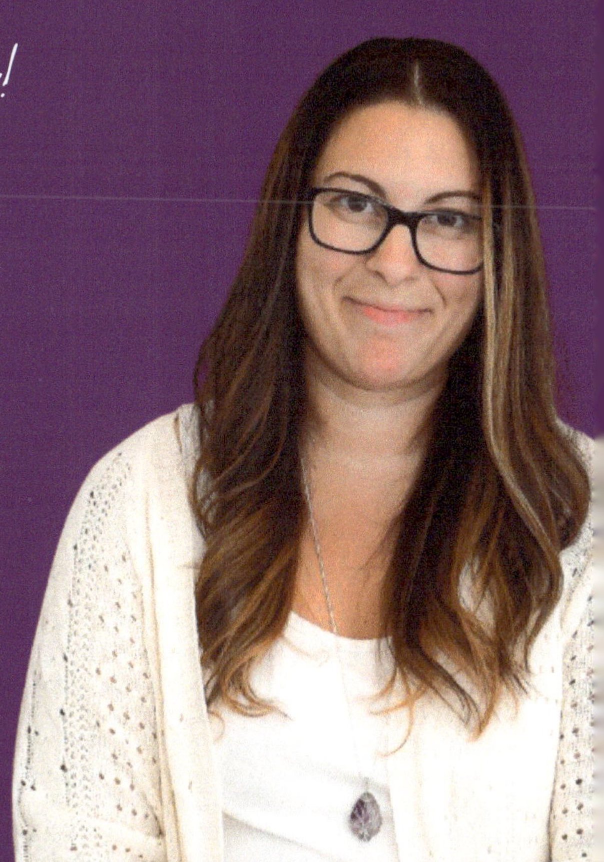

A New Era for Expectant Mothers: The Rise of Prenatal Workouts

By Jordan Searles

One of the biggest and most memorable days of your life has just happened... You're pregnant! With all of the joy and happiness that comes with it, there's unfortunately always unsolicited advice from people who may mean well but are just not up to date on the topic. This especially happens when it comes to pregnancy and exercise.

I was newly pregnant in 2023, and one of my coworkers wanted to stop me from helping him lift a ladder. Knowing my body and my current fitness level, I was more than capable of helping him safely. However, it struck me that there is still this stigma that pregnancy is viewed as a condition or illness where women are meant to take it easy. Thankfully, more and more research is coming out showing that exercise during pregnancy isn't just a 'good idea'; it is crucial for the health of the mother and child.

A common concern I hear from clients regarding exercise and pregnancy is the fear that it will cause a miscarriage. About 10-20% of known pregnancies end in miscarriage, and most miscarriages fall within the first trimester. Some miscarriages have no known cause, while other lifestyle factors are associated with miscarriage. Some of those factors include having a high BMI (30+), a low BMI (<18.5), alcohol consumption during pregnancy, smoking, previous miscarriage, age, uterine abnormalities, and unmanaged illness or disease (such as diabetes, thyroid disease, or polycystic ovarian syndrome). If your lifestyle does not include any of these factors, then exercise during pregnancy would be a very beneficial choice.

One study involving 14,000 women compared those who exercised and those who did not. The group that exercised worked out at a moderate intensity for a maximum of 60 minutes. The findings were that there are 'no associations between volume, intensity, or frequency of exercise and fetal or newborn death' (Davenport, et al. 2019). So rest assured that, as of today, there's no evidence that physical activity increases a woman's risk of miscarriage, preterm birth, or low birth weight. The benefits of exercise for the mother are numerous and may even help with having a better overall experience during pregnancy.

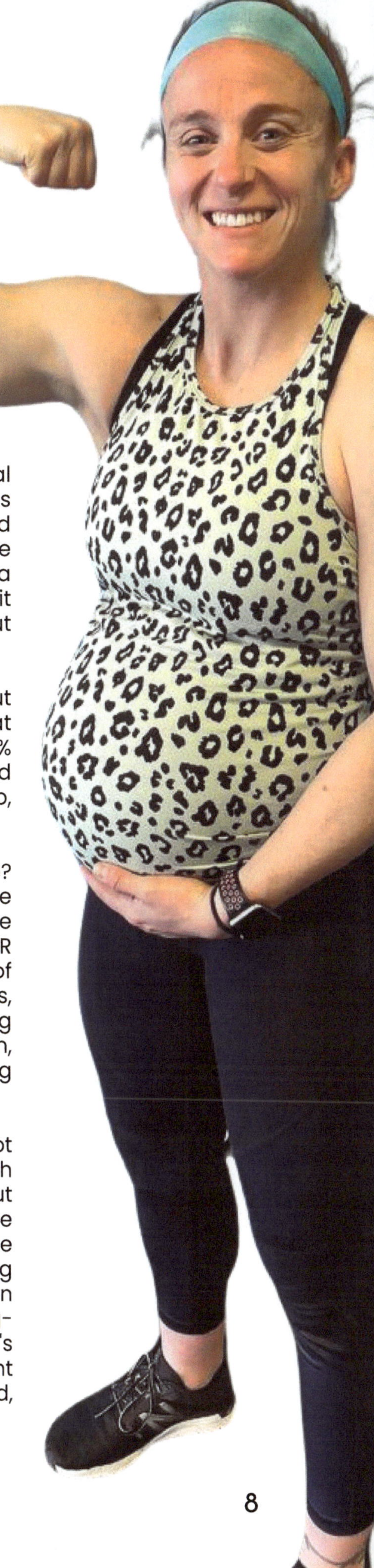

Jordan Searles
Muscle Mama Fitness
NASM CPT Prenatal &
Postpartum Training Specialist
Find her online @jordansrls_fit

Expecting mothers who exercise lower their risk of gestational diabetes, preeclampsia, and some of the other not-so-fun side effects of pregnancy, like nausea, constipation, heartburn, swelling, and varicose veins. It helps minimize excess weight gain outside of the recommended range of 25-35 lbs for single babies. Gaining extra weight can not only be an issue during postpartum recovery, but it also increases the risk of more pain and injuries throughout pregnancy.

There is also a link between women who strength train throughout their pregnancy and their birth experience. A study in 1998 found that those women had a 75% reduction in maternal exhaustion, a 75% reduction in the need for a c-section, and a 50% decrease in the need for medical intervention due to fetal heart-rate abnormalities (Clapp, 1998).

Did you know that babies also benefit from prenatal exercise? Contrary to the belief that mothers who exercise will have premature births or low birth weight babies, exercise actually helps reduce the risk of these outcomes. It is correlated with higher newborn APGAR scores, as well as helping the baby's ability to handle the stress of labor and recover more quickly. Besides these short-term benefits, there have been long-term benefits of prenatal exercise extending into childhood years, such as improved cardiorespiratory health, reducing the risk of childhood obesity, and potentially improving intelligence, language, and memory.

To wrap everything up, the evidence is clear—prenatal exercise is not just beneficial, but critical for the health and well-being of both mother and child. Outdated stigmas and misconceptions about pregnancy as a delicate condition requiring extreme caution are being replaced by a growing understanding of the remarkable resilience and capabilities of the pregnant body. By embracing prenatal workouts tailored to their needs, expectant mothers can experience smoother pregnancies, easier deliveries, and the long-term advantages of fetal programming that supports their child's development. With the right guidance and support, every pregnant woman can go through this journey feeling empowered, not hindered, by the physical demands of carrying new life.

Why is it important for perinatal

Collaboration among perinatal professionals is crucial for providing well-rounded care that meets the diverse needs of mothers. By working together, they can improve health outcomes, offer consistent support, and reduce unnecessary interventions. This teamwork creates a strong support network that empowers mothers, ensuring they feel cared for and confident throughout their pregnancy, birth, and postpartum journey.

Continuing education is a huge part of collaboration and connection. No matter how many years of experience you have, the field is always changing. Standards of care, products, providers, cultural beliefs, are examples. No one can know everything. Connection and knowledge as a village make us stronger as a profession and provide the care women deserve.

This work we do is so solitary to the person providing the support. We learn best in community by shared experiences. It's so important to have a village while doing this work to avoid burnout.

professionals to collaborate?

This way we can see what new things are happening, we can support each other when times get rough. You cannot read everything written about perinatal stats, but together we can all read and share and learn all together.

It is essential for perinatal professionals to connect and collaborate because it allows them to provide comprehensive, well-rounded support to women and mothers during one of the most critical phases of their lives. Collaboration among professionals such as midwives, doulas, lactation consultants, mental health counselors, and obstetricians ensures that care is holistic and addresses the physical, emotional, and psychological needs of women. This multidisciplinary approach not only enhances the quality of care but also helps in identifying and addressing potential issues early on, leading to better health outcomes for both mothers and babies. Moreover, when perinatal professionals work together, they can share knowledge, resources, and best practices, creating a stronger support network for women, which is vital for their overall well-being and empowerment during the perinatal period.

Being able to share experiences we has, the uniqueness of each professional and what they do. Tells us there are more than one way to heal, there are techniques you have always wanted to learn that they teach them. As well as guidance and support from the perinatal professionals. All these can have a huge impact on how you support your clients.

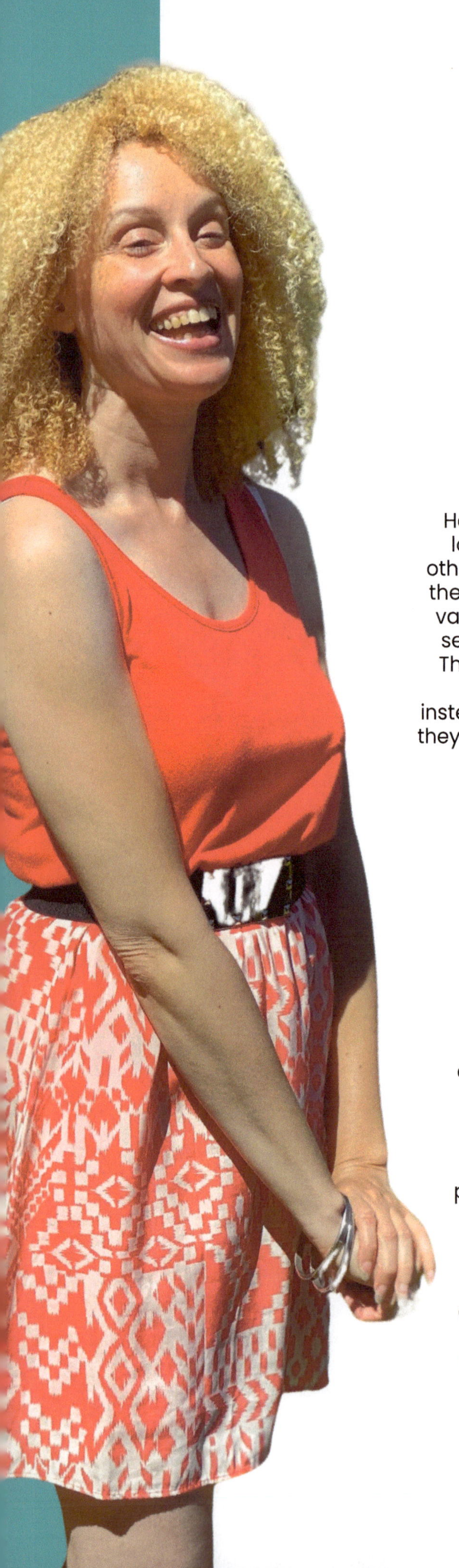

The Importance of Community and Mindfulness

By Khristee Rich

Have you ever stopped to think about the secret to living a long, happy life? In the Blue Zones, people live longer than other parts of the world. Many are centenarians. That's right; they live to be a hundred or more. Their hidden secret? They value community. Friends and family live close by and they see them often. They socialize daily. They walk everywhere. They have hobbies. They cook their own food and use local produce and herbs. They do not use a lot of technology; instead, they do chores by hand, the old-fashioned way, and they spend a lot of time in nature, feel supported, and have a purpose.

Famous biologist and New York Times best-selling author, Dr. Bruce Lipton, says that the key to longevity is not survival of the fittest, but instead it's about living in harmony with nature. He's the Father of Epigenetics, a specialized science that means above genetics. His belief is that we are not victims of our genes but we are creators of our lives and can improve our health outcomes. Simplified, even if our parents developed certain chronic illnesses doesn't mean that we are destined to suffer the same fate. We can change our habits, thoughts, diet, and environment and achieve different results. I, wholeheartedly, believe in the power of community to improve our health and wellness. When we are joyful and relaxed, we feel better. When we can share our hearts and our voices, we feel empowered. Also, I believe we are all creators. We have the power to prevent and overcome illnesses and conditions naturally.

Being in harmony with our natural environment is often overlooked in our wellness journey. So much illness is caused by stress. Western society is not a balanced culture. We yearn for success to our detriment. We forget our humanity. Plus, with technological advances, we risk losing our humanity even more. In 2019, I started working on a three-book series on childbirth around the world through a holistic perspective.

For over twenty years, I have been a healer helping women overcome chronic conditions and illnesses holistically by deciphering the root cause and treating them—mind, body, and spirit—through natural ways and remedies. In my three-book series, I am applying holistic health and wellness to the pregnancy/childbirth journey. To collect case studies, I interviewed about a hundred mothers and childbirth experts. Early in my interviews, I discovered a divide among mothers. There were two distinct sides: those who believed in a medicated birth and those who believed in a non-medicated birth. Views were black and white, with no room in between. Women fought openly with one another. They criticized, judged, and shamed each other. Everyone shared horror stories they had heard from friends, family, doctors, and even strangers, and how these stories tried to influence them to make certain decisions. Moms felt they had to defend themselves from these opinions, especially during pregnancy, when they were most vulnerable.

When I learned about this, I said, 'This is my calling. *I am a healer, and I will bring healing to the subject of childbirth.*' I present childbirth from a holistic view. In my three-book series and in my birth storytelling events, I share childbirth stories to bring understanding of why chronic conditions happen in pregnancy and postpartum, why birth complications occur, and how they can be prevented and treated naturally. The stories are real and complex, demonstrating that childbirth is individual, not black and white, and that the whole journey is essential—from pregnancy (sometimes conception) through postpartum. I emphasize the importance of doulas throughout the journey, from pregnancy through postpartum. This support helps women emotionally, physically, and spiritually, and can minimize the risks of developing health conditions, having traumatic births, or feeling ill-prepared. It's also important to note that I highlight the significance of preparing for childbirth in preconception instead of during pregnancy, so women can make informed decisions and improve their health and wellness to minimize the development of chronic conditions in pregnancy and postpartum, birth complications, and unhealthy children. I believe this information will unify women. We don't need to be divided. The outcomes of childbirth are more complex than are realized in a short story, which is only about decisions at birth and not about a mother's prior health before pregnancy, her health during pregnancy and postpartum, her baby's health in utero, and more. Mindfulness is so important. I am creating fresh birth storytelling. I believe knowledge and understanding in preconception from a holistic perspective will help mothers and moms-to-be dissolve this invisible divide among women.

I believe we all want the same thing: to be healthy, to thrive, to be seen and heard, to have a healthy baby, and to have no regrets. The good news is that even if we don't live in the Blue Zones, we can still take conscious action to be more social, build our community, prioritize our health, have fun, be present in nature, relax, and strive to overcome our illnesses to live longer, richer lives— even during the pregnancy/childbirth journey. We can still strive to live the values that matter to us. We need the support of our local and extended community. There are so many perinatal professionals with a wealth of knowledge and talents to assist women. But not only do mothers need a robust community, so do perinatal professionals. We are stronger as a village.

Khristee Rich

The Dancing Curtain LLC
Writer, Healer, Speaker
Find her online @khristeerich
www.thedancingcurtain.com

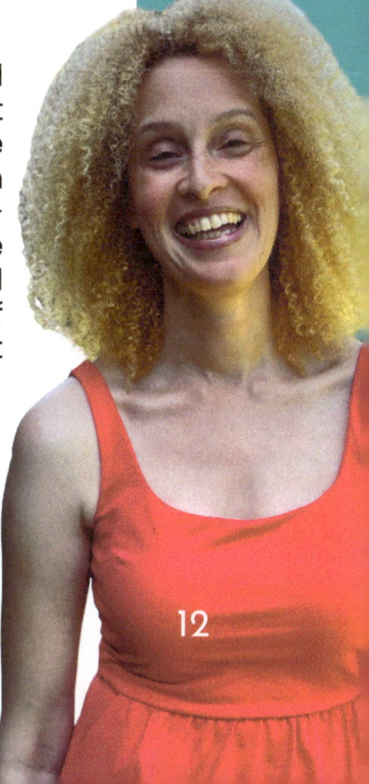

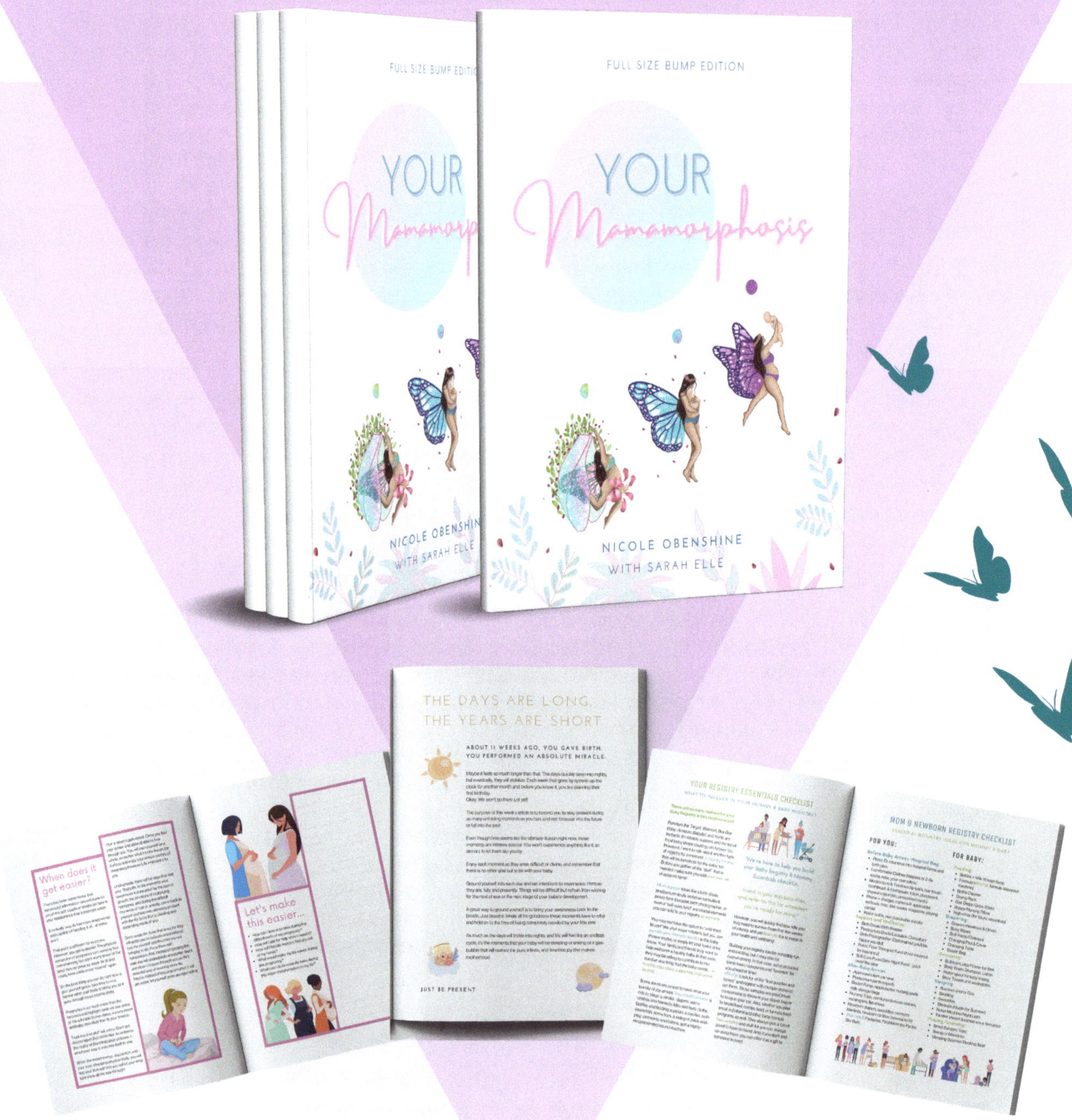

Get access to articles for all four trimesters, supportive journal prompts, birth and postpartum plan templates, a space for your birth story, an affirmation poster, and real experiences and stories from moms. This tangible resource for your journey is available for *only $10.*

SCAN QR CODE TO PURCHASE

FLOWCODE PRIVACY.FLOWCODE.COM

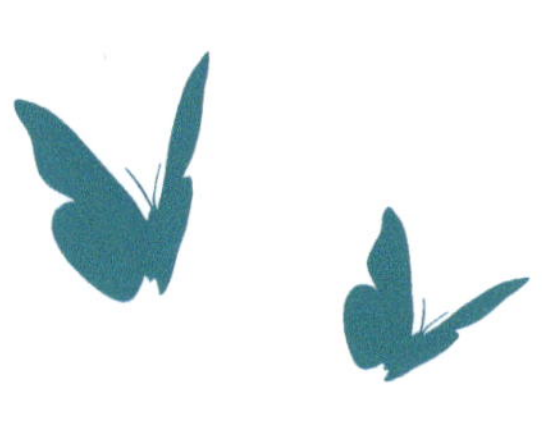

How to Be a Consumer During Your Pregnancy

By Amy Bauer

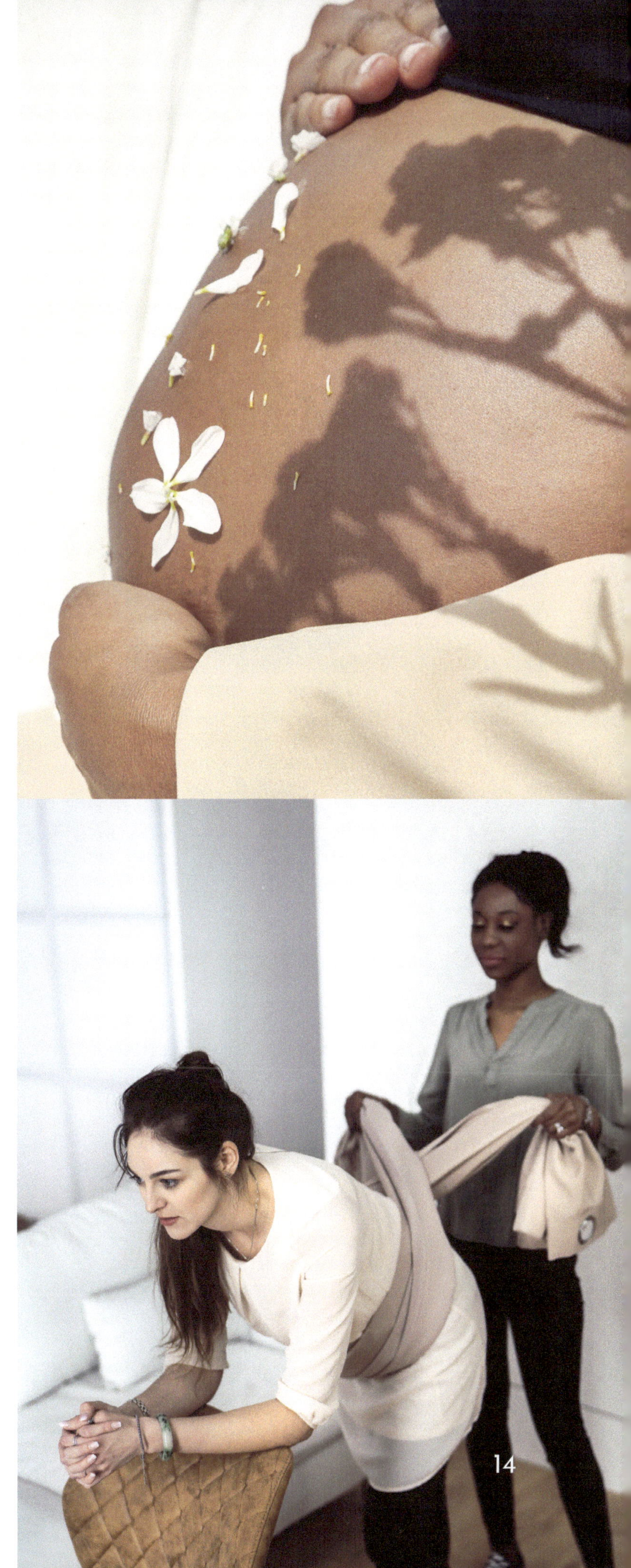

Have you ever thought about how much time goes into planning a wedding? How about a big party? Many hours of research and planning may be involved in looking into a house you were thinking of buying or a neighborhood that you are considering moving to.   But how much time to most women spend thinking about how they want their birth to go? Much of the time little, if any, thought goes into what type of birth a woman would like to have or what plans need to be set in place to achieve it. But, like anything else in life, your satisfaction with the outcome of your birth will be directly influenced by the amount of preparation and consideration given beforehand. Now, it is true, that birth cannot be "planned" in a certain sense. After all, we only have so much control over how things happen. Nevertheless, there are always things that you can do in advance to give yourself the best path forward for "success" ...however you define that. And regardless of what the ultimate outcome is, you will be able to rest in the knowledge that you did all in your power to achieve your ideal birth and protect yourself and your baby. You will be able to look back on your birth experience with a sense of agency and no regrets.

In this article we will explore the four essential steps to becoming a consumer in the birth world.

01

REMEMBER WHO YOU ARE

This may seem obvious and like it doesn't need to be said, but think about it for just one moment. In the scenario of birth, you are an employer! Say that out loud to yourself: 'I am the employer.' And who is it exactly that you are employing? Well, first and foremost, your doctor or midwife. Secondly, the hospital or birth center where you are delivering. And perhaps also a doula. In each of those instances, you are in the driver's seat.

Now, I realize that in our system, we use other words. For example, the word 'patient' sets an entirely different tone for the transaction that you are engaging in. But think of the wider world. In what scenario do you go anywhere, pay someone for services you require of them, and then they tell you what you must do? Nowhere else do we find this strange dynamic where the person paying for a service finds themselves in a position of being told what they are 'allowed' or 'required' to do.

It may be true that you are hiring these clinicians because they are more knowledgeable in the area of birth than you are. But the fact remains that, at the end of the day, they are consultants. YOU are the project manager. They may give you advice, but it is up to you whether you take it or whether you decide to go a different way. It is absolutely within your rights to question their advice, to ask them to defend it, or to ignore it and do something different.

Your doctor or midwife should absolutely inform you of problems or risks they see in your path, but only you and your partner are qualified to determine which risks you choose to assume. No one should be forcing you to assume risks that they think are best for you. Now that you are firmly grounded in who you are, we move on to:

02

SET YOUR PRIORITIES

This is an important next step in moving forward because step three is to hire the right people.

But how are you going to know who the right people are if you are not sure of what the goals are? That would be like setting out on a journey without knowing your destination. I think we have already established that the foundational goal is the survival of all parties involved. But as for the specific goals, well, those are going to be as many and varied as the women who are setting them.

For some women, the goal is to have a stress-free birth where they don't have to make many decisions and do not have to experience the pain of childbirth. Their priorities might be that their doctor is very personable and has a great bedside manner. For other women, the goal is to have a very 'hands-off' birth with as few interventions as possible. Those women may want to hire a midwife.

Or it may be that a woman's priorities are not super set in stone, but the primary goal is to avoid a surgical birth. These women may want to look for a doctor or midwife, but they will want both the clinical providers and the hospital they choose to have a lower-than-average c-section rate.

In some cases, a woman might have an aversion to hospitals, and if she is healthy and low risk, she may feel like her highest priority is to give birth in her own space, and so she chooses a home birth with a qualified midwife. But in all cases, it is necessary to know what is most important to you BEFORE you move on to the next step.

HIRE THE RIGHT PEOPLE

Now, here is where things get a little trickier. As we all know, the way our system is set up, we often do not feel that we have as much say in these matters as we would like. For example, we let our insurance coverage dictate who our provider choices are, and then we just try to make the best choice we feel is available to us. This can make us feel limited or even trapped. But I want to give you a few things to think about. Let's go back to looking at how other transactions go. When you go to build a house, you do not necessarily want to pick the cheapest builder just because he is the cheapest. The reason we may be willing to pay more is that we feel the quality of the work is worth the cost. Hiring a doctor is no different. The problem with our system of maternity 'care' is that becoming a doctor doesn't automatically mean they are a good doctor. So, choosing a doctor based on the options your insurance company offers may not always be the best option.

Ask yourself: If I end up with a surgical birth because I was bullied into making decisions I wasn't comfortable with, am I going to be happy with this hire? Remember step 1: you are the employer.
Also, asking for recommendations isn't necessarily the best route either—unless you know that the person you are asking has the same basic priorities as you do. Are you going to be glad that your doctor was friendly and personable if you feel they did not listen to you, include you in decision-making for your care, or respect your desires? So, I am going to advise you to do your research with regard to the hospital and clinical care provider that you choose. This is one of the most important factors in the ultimate outcome of your birth. Take a look at how different the rates of surgical birth can be from one hospital to another and from one doctor to another, and you will quickly see that there is no one standard of care.

KNOW THE DIFFERENCE

Agreeing to go along with a doctor's advice is consent... but it is not necessarily informed consent. Informed consent is when a patient is fully educated about the risks, benefits, and alternatives of a given procedure or intervention. Often in the realm of birth, things are not presented this way at all. It is much more common for patients to be told how things are going to be done. Many times, this is based on the conveniences of the clinical provider or on hospital policies that have little, if anything, to do with what works well for the patient and much more to do with what makes the most sense for the hospital or doctor.

When I was pregnant with my first baby, I have a vivid memory of naively asking my OB when we would talk about my options for birth. Her response is one I will never forget. She said, '*What options?*' Knowing that you have the right to informed consent and understanding that things are unlikely to be presented to you this way gives you the permission you may need to question the advice you are being given, to ask for alternatives, and to understand that just because advice is given to you, doesn't mean you have to take it. It also doesn't mean that going another way would be unreasonable—although you may experience pushback from clinical providers who are not accustomed to being questioned, let alone refused. Hospital policies are not laws. Standing orders are not commands that you must obey. Further, it isn't even common for decisions made during birth to be emergent... so usually it is very reasonable to ask for time. Time to process what is happening and to evaluate what you truly want to do. And if you do have to accept outcomes that are not what you wanted, at the very least, you deserve time to come to terms with things, rather than feeling like everything is out of control and being forced on you.

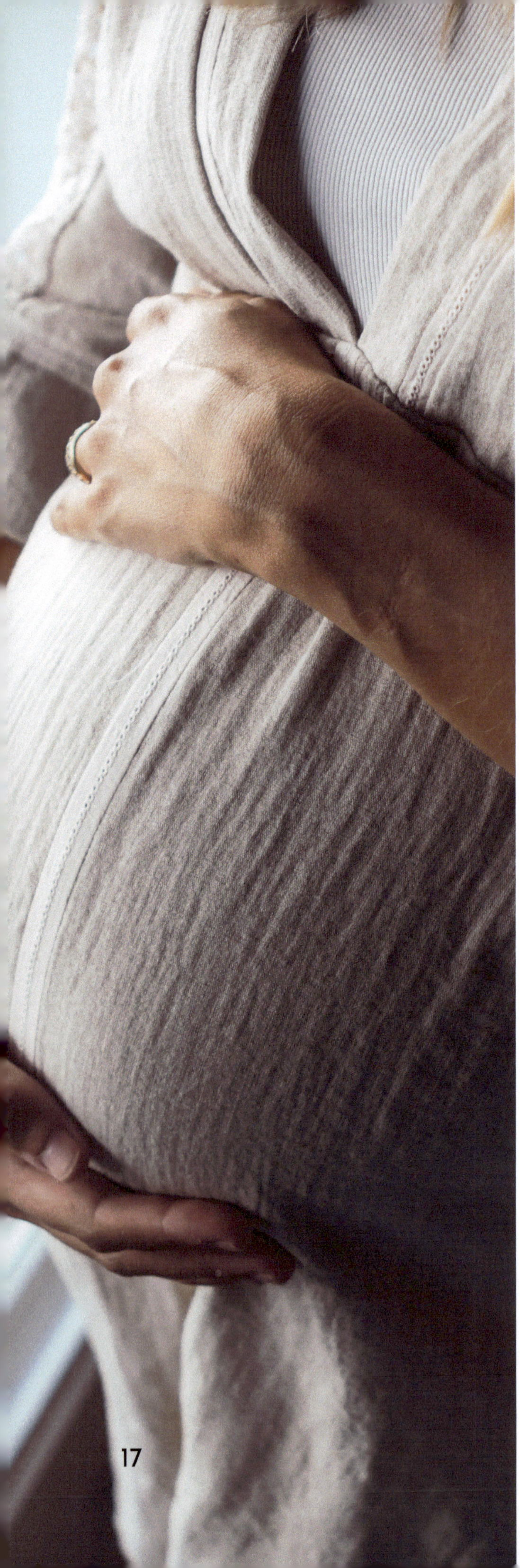

Lastly, keep in mind that there really is no substitute for *hiring a doula* to attend your birth.

If this has given you some things to think about with regard to being a consumer in your birth experience, then it has been a success.

Remember, doctors and midwives don't "deliver" babies. Doctors and midwives catch the babies that are delivered by their patients.

Your birth experience does not have to be something that a broken system imposes on you. Take it back. **Own it. It belongs to you, and it is too precious to have it stolen from you**.

The changes that really need to happen within our maternity care system will only begin to unfold when a majority of women realize this and walk gracefully and confidently into that reality. It may be a bit more work, but the quality and value of the outcome of that effort will be something that you will never regret.

Amy Bauer
Owner, *Hoosier Doula Network*
Creator of *Pocket Doula,*

Certified Doula, and Childbirth Educator
Find her online @hoosierdoulanetwork
and at www.hoosierdoula.net

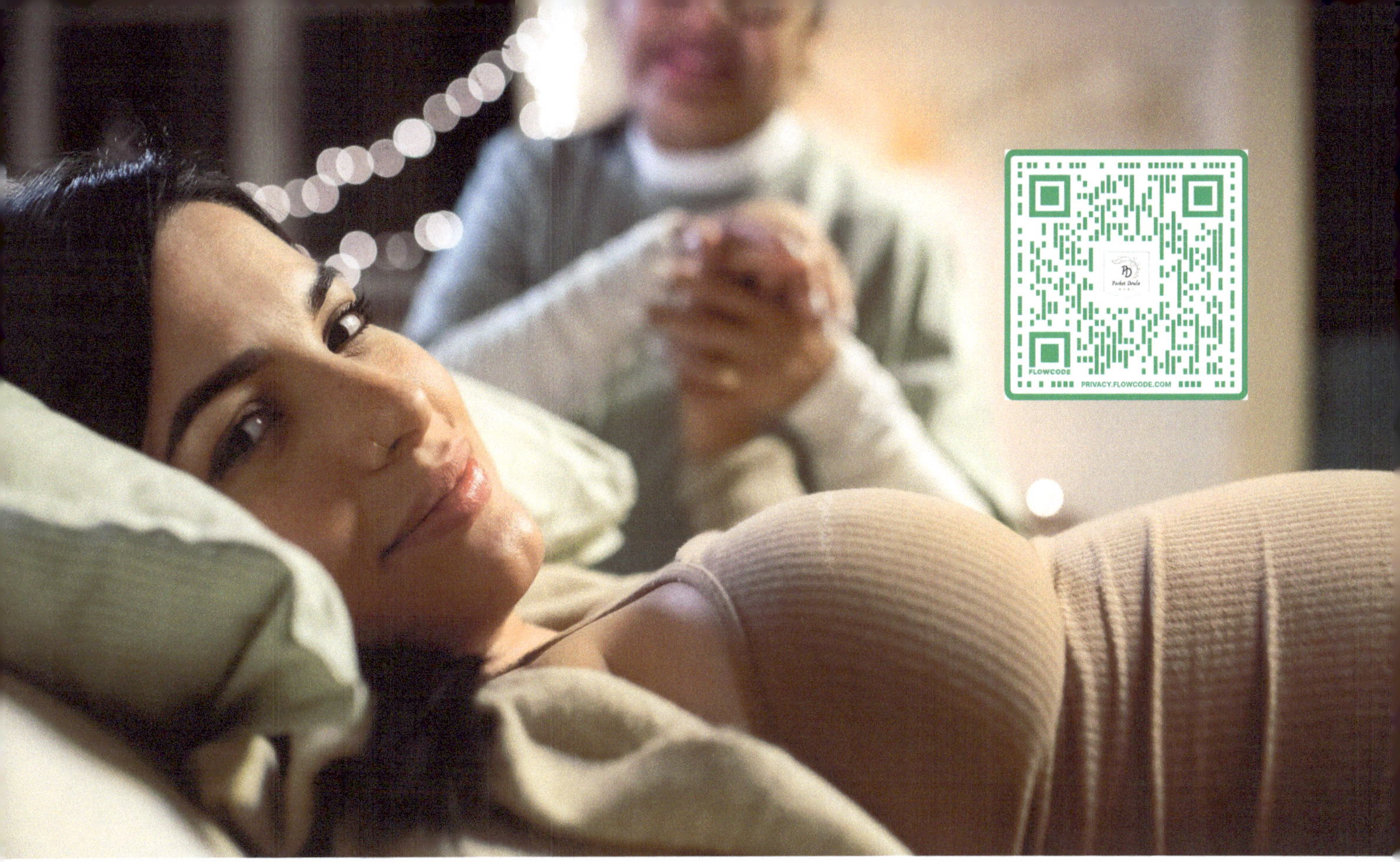

In-person doulas are an invaluable resource for navigating your ideal birth. But the help a doula provides isn't all at go-time. A large percentage of the value of a doula comes from all the information and resources she provides to you prior to your labor. But what if you had that information at your fingertips… even right in your own pocket? Now you can!

Hoosier Doula is excited to introduce to you our new app: **Pocket Doula.** Whether it's practicing relaxation techniques, looking for suggestions for which position to use and when, or trying to remember what you learned in your childbirth education class, Pocket Doula makes utilizing your resources as easy as pulling out your phone and looking at our app. Suggestions for how to take back your birth, avoid birth trauma, and evaluate risk. Connect with other moms in our Pocket Doula Community to support one another.

Look for future classes and resources coming soon, such as Postpartum Tips and Tricks, Help with Breastfeeding and Newborn Care, and much, much more. Get Pocket Doula and take learning and support for your pregnancy journey with you wherever you go!

Scan the QR code to visit our website and go to the Apple or Google Play store to download today!

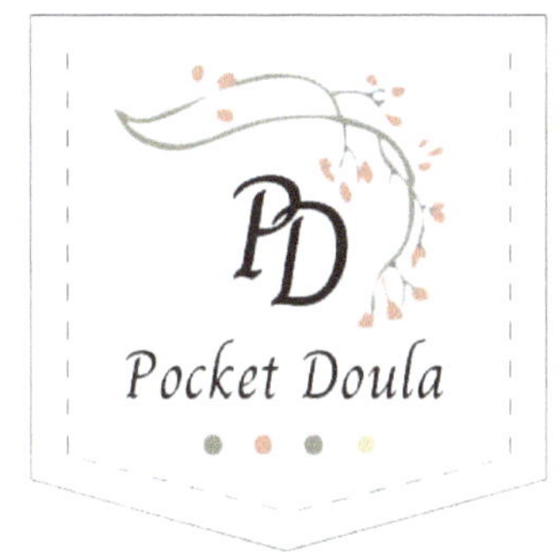

HOW TO ASK FOR SUPPORT

From Your Partner

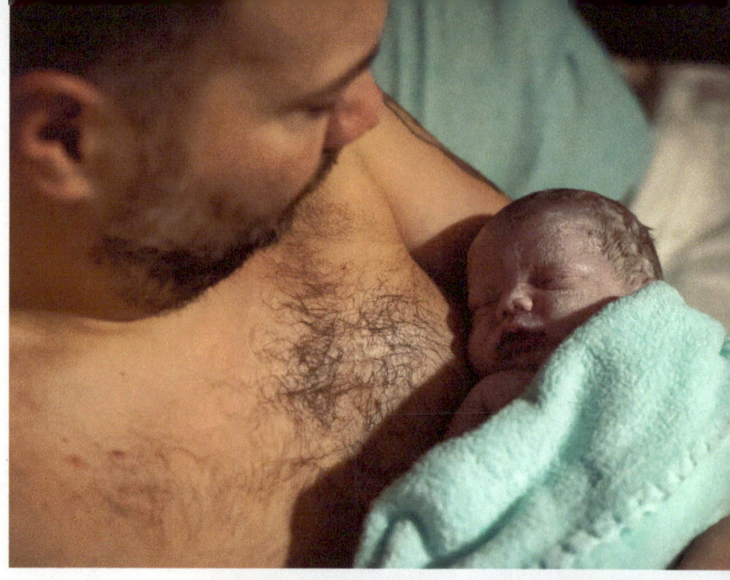

Many of us during the perinatal period have certain wants, needs, boundaries, preferences, or other aspects that we hope to communicate during pregnancy in preparation to our birth and postpartum. And likely the person who hears those the most is our partner. However, regardless of if they *hear you, are they really listening and understanding what you are needing and wanting. This article will give you some tips to ensure your values and expectations are communicated appropriately and not ignored, dismissed or misunderstood.*

Your partners typically have the best intentions but may respond in a way that comes from fear, uncertainty, or other narratives that are influencing their ability to see your view. The best way for them to support us, is for us to support them in understanding the basic what, when, where, how, who and why questions. Additionally, they need to understand that birth is an investment, just like a wedding or home purchase. They should have the same level of financial fluidity for birth as they do for those other events.

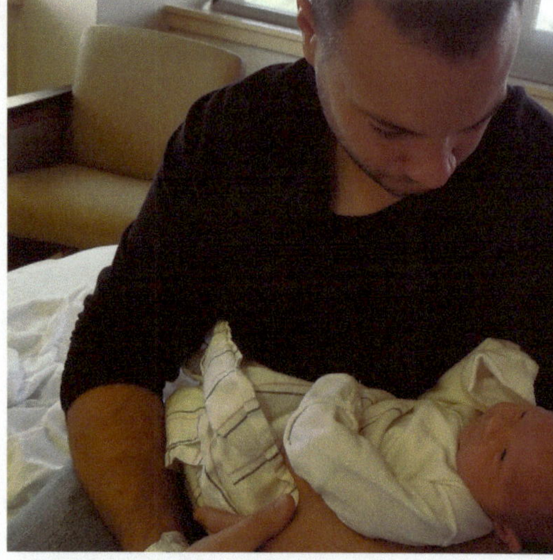

By Nicole Harlot

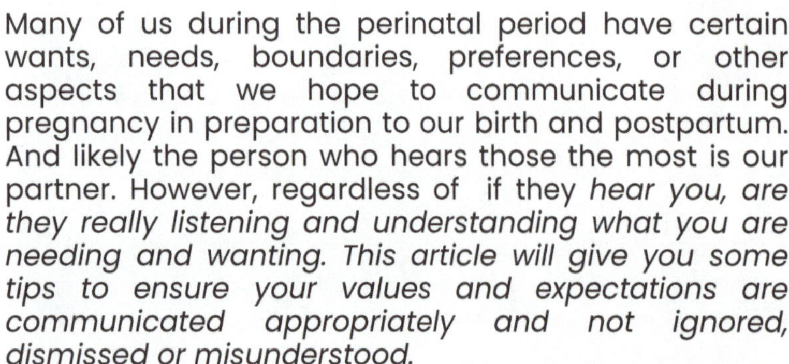

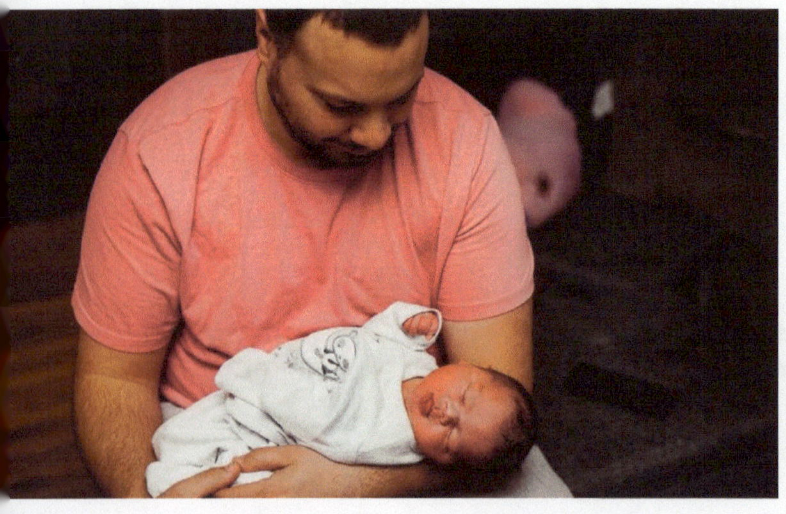

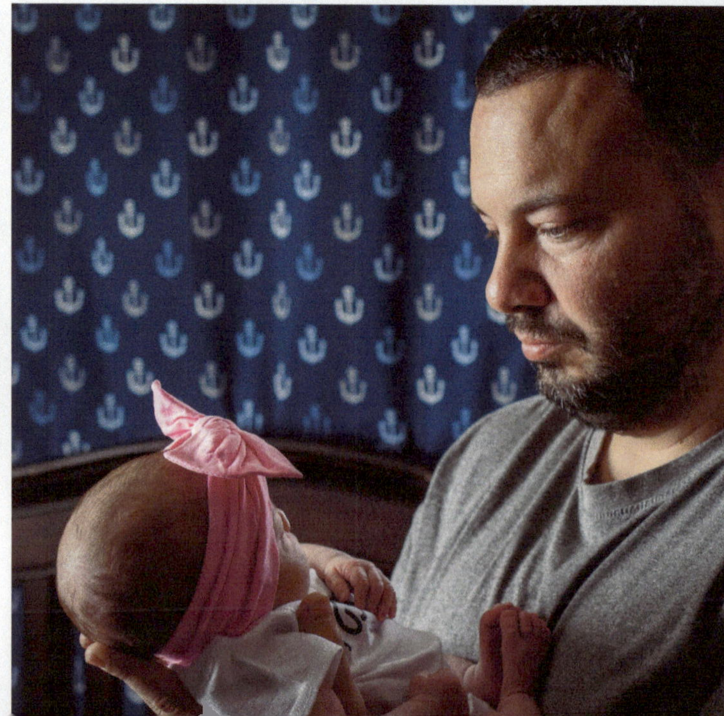

THE BASIC QUESTIONS

WHAT?

what are your preferences, what do you want your birth to look like, what do you need to feel educated, safe and empowered, what can he do to support you when you are in labor, what can he do to support you in postpartum.

WHERE?

Where do you want to labor, where do you want to birth, where do you want yourself set up in those few days after baby arrives?

WHEN?

When should he step in, when should he advocate for what you want, when should you call the doctor, when should you call your support team, when do you want visitors, when do you want others to hold the baby.

WHO?

Who do you want present at your birth, who do you NOT want present, who do you want on your support team, who do you want to visit the hospital, or home once you are there. Who is your "go to" person if you are not feeling well in postpartum?

HOW?

How can he help you in labor, how can he make it more peaceful, how can he advocate when he needs to because you are in your body in active labor, how can he best prepare the house and meals for postpartum. Not just WHAT but HOW is important.

WHY?

Why do these things matter to you, why is it important to discuss beforehand and not during or after, why is it necessary for you to communicate all of this to him/her specifically.

Set time aside in your second or third trimester for you and your partner to have a serious conversation about labor, birth and postpartum. It is important that they feel informed and empowered for what YOU want, and not be combative in situations that may seem scary or uncertain.

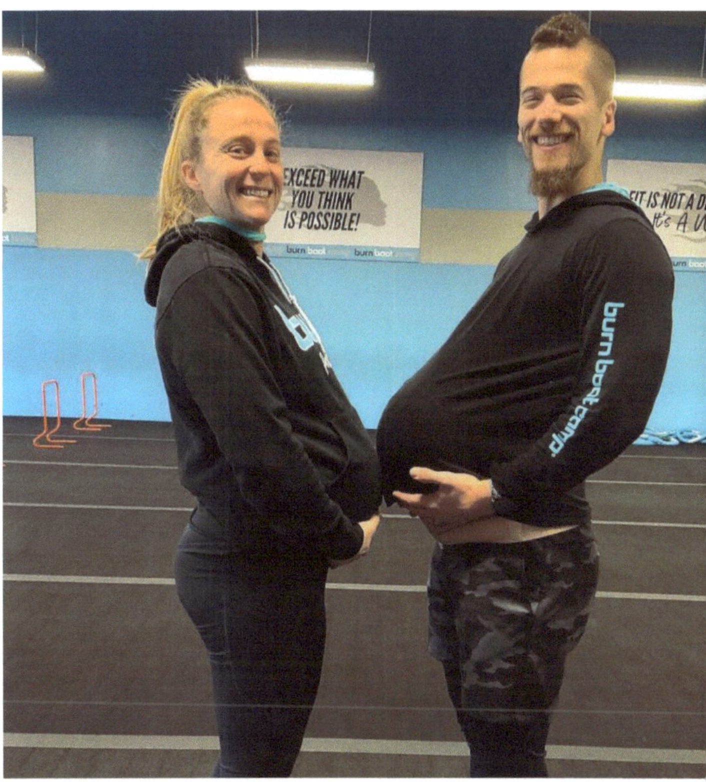

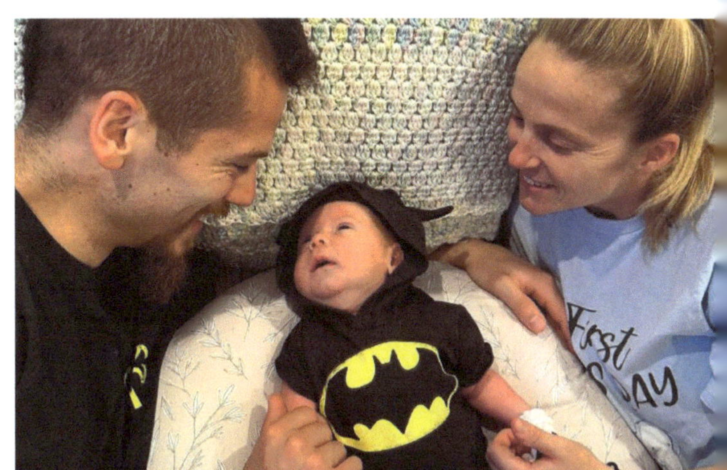

Cervical Scar Tissue: Recognizing a Hidden Cause of Unnecessary C-Sections and How to Advocate for Yourself

By Dawn Thompson

Dawn Thompson is a seasoned birth professional with over 20 years of experience in the field. As the founder of Birthify, she is a passionate advocate for maternal health and has dedicated her career to improving birth outcomes through education, awareness, and support. Dawn is widely recognized for her pioneering work on cervical scar tissue, having written the first article on the subject in 2009, which sparked global awareness and discussion. Her commitment to empowering women and challenging the status quo continues to inspire both her clients and the broader birth community.

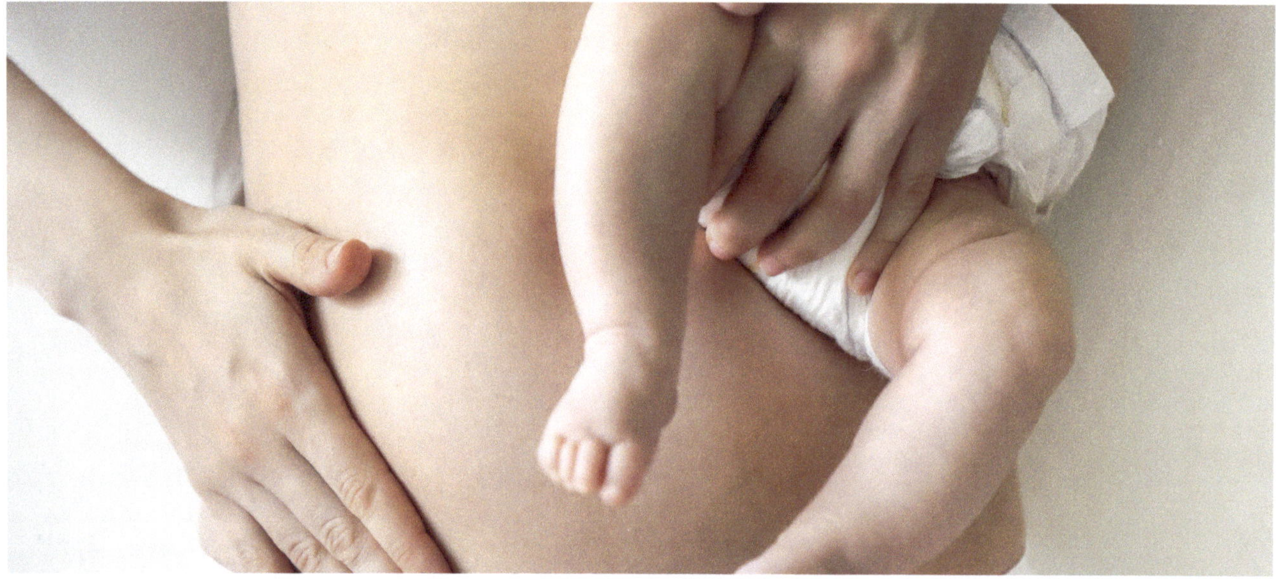

In 2006, as a dedicated birth professional, I first encountered a term that would change the course of my career and impact countless lives: cervical scar tissue. At the time, it was an issue that no one was talking about—a hidden cause behind many so-called "failure to progress" diagnoses that often led to unnecessary C-sections.

After years of reflecting on this and seeing its implications in my work, I wrote an article in 2009 titled *Cervical Scar Tissue – A Big Issue That No One Is Talking About*. This became the first article on the internet to address this critical topic. The response was overwhelming. The article went viral, resonating with women and birth professionals worldwide, and has since been read by countless people. It inspired many birth professionals to write about cervical scar tissue, and it began to be taught in doula and midwifery programs across the country. Unfortunately, to my knowledge, it still hasn't reached medical training programs, where the majority of providers assisting in pregnancies in the U.S. are educated. This means the issue remains significant if no one asks the right questions or considers this possibility.

21

Understanding Cervical Scar Tissue

Cervical scar tissue, or cervical stenosis, can develop after procedures like LEEP, Cone, Cryo, D&C, or even IUD placement. These procedures often involve the use of a cervical stabilizer (Tenaculum), which can pierce the cervix and lead to scarring. This scarring can impede the cervix's ability to dilate appropriately during labor, resulting in a stalled labor often diagnosed as "failure to progress." Without recognizing the presence of scar tissue, many healthcare providers may recommend interventions, including unnecessary C-sections.

Recognizing the Signs of Cervical Scar Tissue

If you're pregnant or planning a pregnancy, being aware of the signs of cervical scar tissue is crucial. Here are some key indicators:

- **Prodromal Labor:** You experience labor-like contractions over days or weeks, but they don't lead to active labor.
- **Dilation Stall:** Despite strong contractions, your cervix dilates slowly or not at all.
- **High Effacement, Low Dilation:** Your cervix becomes very thin (high effacement), but the dilation remains minimal.
- **Urge to Push with Low Dilation:** You feel an overwhelming urge to push, but your cervix hasn't dilated enough.

How to Advocate for Yourself

Understanding cervical scar tissue is just the first step. Here's how you can advocate for yourself if you suspect cervical scar tissue might impact your birth:

- **Educate Yourself and Your Partner:** Knowledge is power. Ensure you and your partner understand cervical scar tissue, its causes, and its implications.
- **Know Your Rights:** You have the right to ask for time and avoid rushed decisions during labor. If labor stalls, inquire whether scar tissue could be a factor before agreeing to interventions like a C-section.

- **Talk to Your Healthcare Provider:** Discuss your concerns with your healthcare provider early in your pregnancy. Share your medical history, especially any procedures that could have caused cervical scarring. Ask if they are familiar with cervical scar tissue and how they would manage it during labor.
- **Consider a Second Opinion:** If your provider seems unaware or dismissive of cervical scar tissue, consider seeking a second opinion, preferably from a midwife or ObGyn experienced in VBACs or natural birth.
- **Prepare for Labor:** If you're at risk, discuss possible interventions with your provider, such as manual massage of the cervix to break up scar tissue during labor.
- **Hire a Doula:** A doula experienced in VBACs and cervical scar tissue can provide invaluable support and advocacy during labor.

Moving Forward

As we continue to raise awareness, it's crucial for women to be informed and prepared to advocate for themselves. By understanding the signs of cervical scar tissue and how to address it, you can help avoid unnecessary interventions and experience the birth you deserve—one that is informed, supported, and free from preventable complications.

Your voice matters in this conversation, and by speaking up, you can help bring about the change needed to ensure that cervical scar tissue is recognized and treated appropriately in all births. Together, we can ensure that every woman has the opportunity to have a safe and empowering birth experience.

Dawn Thompson
Birthify
Virtual Doula Support, Full Spectrum Doula, Speaker, Writer, Advocate
Find her on social media @birthify_

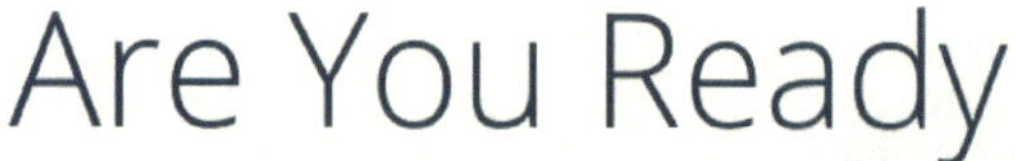

Are You Ready

For a Smoother Birth and Postpartum Experience?

Finally, the Support Every New Parent Has Always Needed

Scan Me

- **Full-spectrum doula care for pregnancy, birth, postpartum, and newborn care**

- **Available 24/7 through messaging and virtual coaching**

- **More affordable than traditional doula services**

- **Get answers to questions you didn't know to ask**

www.birthify.net

23

Beyond the Bounce Back: De-Commercializing Postpartum Care & Reclaiming the Village

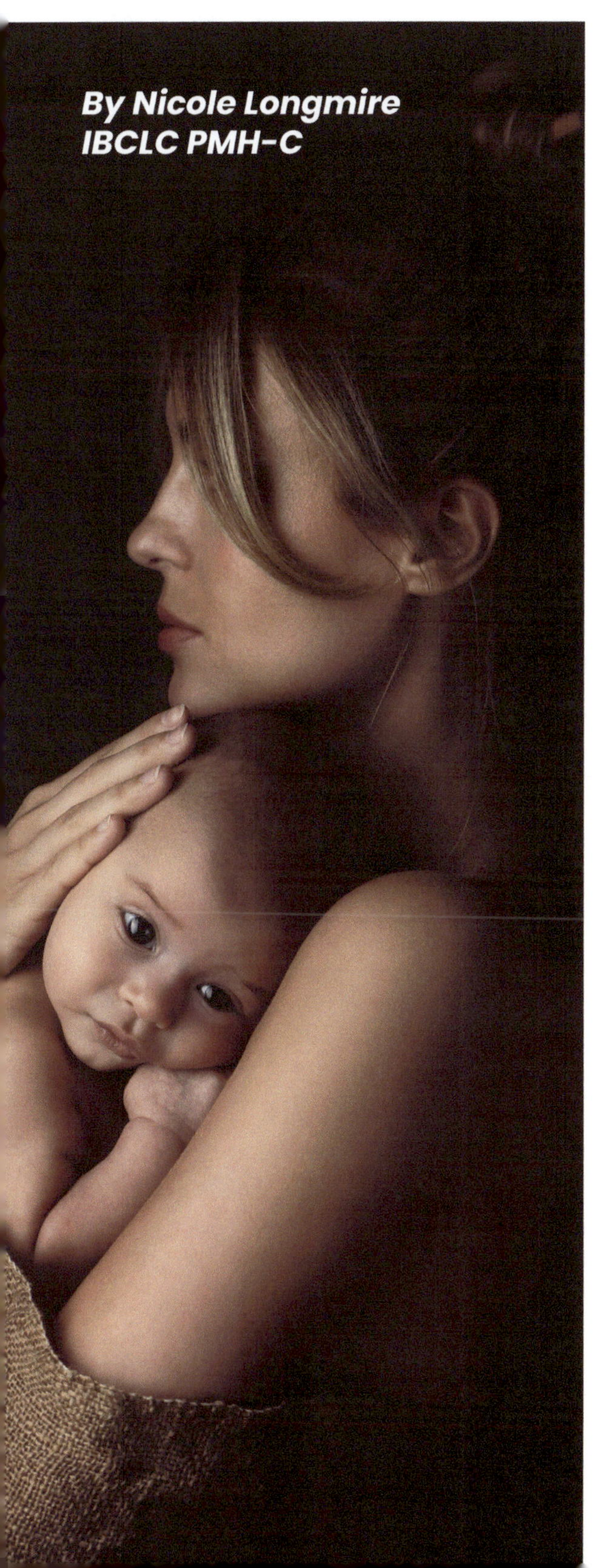

The loss of the "village" — referring to the traditional social support system of extended families and close-knit communities — has significantly impacted many aspects of parenting, especially women in the early postpartum period.

History and Importance of the Village

Historically, women received guidance, encouragement, and hands-on help from experienced mothers, grandmothers, aunts, and other community members, which facilitated the transition to motherhood and allowed for natural process to occur (like bonding with her baby, caring for herself, recovering from birth, the identify and emotional changes and shifts, the natural breastfeeding process, and infant care). The absence of this village and subsequent consequences of it has lead to a significant breakdown in the natural development of women; in some ways, akin to a child not being neglected and thus being "stunted" developmentally. This neglect of mothers can have both immediate and long-term consequences, potentially stunting their physical, emotional, and psychological development across the lifespan.

Without proper support—whether it be through family help, healthcare services, or communal care—women may struggle to rest, heal, and transition emotionally to their new role. This lack of care can lead to chronic issues, such as pelvic floor disorders, ongoing pain, fatigue, and even complications from untreated physical trauma. Postpartum depression and anxiety may develop or worsen in such an environment, with little emotional support or validation for the challenges they face. Neglecting emotional support during this time can strain relationships, leading to feelings of resentment or detachment from partners or loved ones. Additionally, a mother's emotional health directly affects her ability to bond with her baby, which can impact the child's development, emotional security, and social skills in the long term. Without adequate support, new mothers are at an increased risk of developing postpartum depression (PPD), anxiety, or even postpartum psychosis.

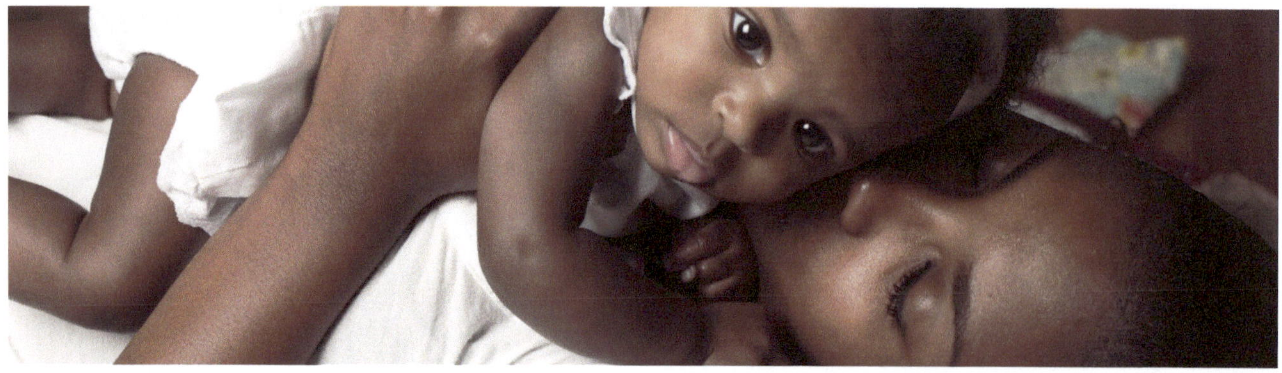

The pressure to manage alone can exacerbate mental health issues, which, if left untreated, can persist well beyond the postpartum period and affect a woman's ability to cope with life's challenges. Mental health challenges that begin in the postpartum period can have long-term consequences, contributing to chronic anxiety, depression, or other psychological disorders. This can affect a woman's self-esteem, her relationships, and her overall quality of life for many years to come. Additionally, maternal mortality review committees report that over 60% of U.S. maternal deaths may have been prevented with more timely diagnoses and effective treatment for postpartum onset conditions, as well as improved patient knowledge of warning signs. The majority of maternal deaths occur in the 42 days following birth with approximately 25% occurring after women are discharged from the hospital following pregnancies and deliveries that appear uncomplicated.

This lack of postpartum support is part of a broader societal pattern that undervalues caregiving and maternal health. It is also reflective of broader systemic failures, such as inadequate maternity leave policies, poor access to healthcare, and a lack of affordable childcare. This neglect is compounded by societal expectations that mothers should "bounce back" quickly and manage both motherhood and other responsibilities with little outside help.

The Commercialization of Postpartum Care

In response to this crisis, we have seen an uptick in the commercialization of postpartum care, which refers to the process by which the care and support that new mothers need during the postpartum period has been turned into a profitable business. I

Instead of viewing postpartum care as a community or family responsibility, modern societies, especially in capitalist economies, often treat it as a product or service that can be bought. This shift commodifies essential care and promotes the idea that mothers should purchase solutions for their physical and emotional recovery.

The commercialization of postpartum care shifts the responsibility of recovery from a communal effort to an individual one. Mothers are often told that they can "buy" their way to better health, comfort, or mental well-being, an approach that encourages mothers to see their recovery as their own responsibility, isolating them from the communal support that was once integral to postpartum care.

This serves to reinforce the notion that postpartum recovery is something that can and should be managed alone with the right purchases, and stands in contrast to the idea of communal care, where support is shared and given freely within families and communities. The push for mothers to rely on commercial services for care often stigmatizes the idea of asking for help from friends, family, or community members. This can further isolate mothers, making them feel like they should be able to handle everything on their own with the right products, rather than fostering an environment where asking for and receiving help is normalized.

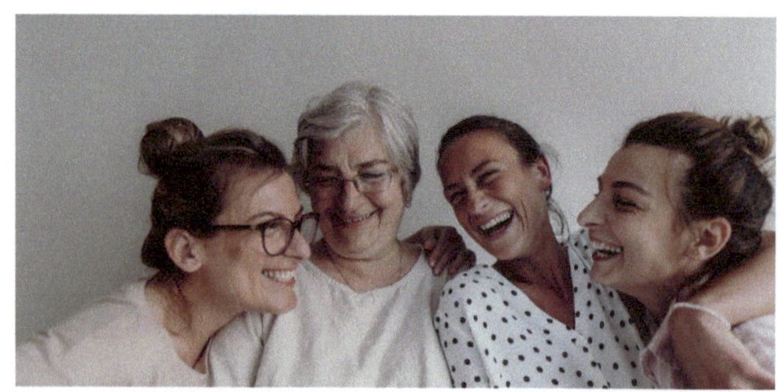

One example of commercialized postpartum care is the focus on "self care." Telling postpartum moms they need self-care, while often well-intentioned, can sometimes be unhelpful or even counterproductive for several reasons. Telling a new mom she needs self-care places the burden of her well-being solely on her, without addressing the external factors that contribute to her stress, exhaustion, or mental health struggles. Simply telling them to practice self-care can feel dismissive of the enormity of their responsibilities. It can lead to feelings of inadequacy or guilt if the mother feels unable to find time for self-care, adding more pressure rather than relieving it.

It is also a gross over-simplification of the postpartum person and the needs of this period. The postpartum period is complex, involving emotional, physical, and mental adjustments. Suggesting that self-care will solve these challenges can oversimplify what new mothers actually need. Often, they need practical support, such as help with household chores, childcare, or emotional support from family, friends, or professionals, rather than the message that they should find time for a bath or a manicure.

The concept of "self-care" has deep roots in historical movements, particularly those centered around collective resistance and empowerment, but it has been increasingly co-opted and commodified in recent years. This transformation, often referred to as the colonization of self-care, shifts the focus from its original political and collective meaning to a more individualistic and commercialized form. Over time, the concept of self-care has been "colonized" by consumerism, wellness industries, and capitalist systems, diluting its original meaning and transforming it into a marketable, individualistic practice. This commodification prioritizes consumption over the original, community-centered ideals, suggesting that self-care can be "bought" rather than being about survival or collective healing. This self-centered version of self-care, which is often promoted on social media, tends to ignore or obscure the structural causes of postpartum depletion, postpartum mental health disorders, low breastfeeding rates, and even poor infant mental health; such as systemic inequality, discrimination, and lack of social support.

The Role of Perinatal Professionals:

As perinatal professionals, helping to decolonize self-care, de-commercialize postpartum, and revive the concept of "the village" requires a collective approach that challenges individualistic and commercialized notions of self-care while fostering a community-based support system for postpartum women.

 Within each of our spheres of influence, there are subtle shifts we can make that can move the needle. Some simple suggestions are things like offering to take out the trash when you leave from a home visit, or folding the laundry on her couch while providing education on postpartum recovery. As perinatal professionals, we play a pivotal role by fostering community-based, accessible, and culturally competent approaches to postpartum care. By working together and shifting the focus away from individual responsibility toward collective care, we can build the "village" around new mothers, offering them the practical, emotional, and mental support they truly need.

1. Reframe Self-Care as Collective Care:

- **Educate and Communicate:** Shift the language of self-care from an individual responsibility to one that involves community support. When interacting with postpartum mothers, emphasize that self-care doesn't need to be something they do alone but should be a collaborative effort that involves family, friends, and healthcare professionals.
- **Encourage Collective Practices:** Promote the idea that postpartum recovery and well-being require the support of others. This could mean encouraging partners, family members, and friends to be actively involved in caring for the mother, not just the baby.

2. Promote Community Support Systems:

- **Create or Support Peer Groups:** Help facilitate peer support groups where women can come together, share experiences, and offer mutual aid. These groups provide emotional, mental, and practical support, which is crucial during the postpartum period. Connecting women with others in similar situations fosters a sense of community and shared responsibility.
- **Leverage Local Resources:** Link mothers to local networks, such as postpartum support organizations, parent groups, or community health programs, which can provide resources ranging from lactation support to mental health services.

3. Advocate for Systemic Changes:

- **Address Socioeconomic and Structural Barriers:** Recognize that not all women have the same access to traditional forms of "self-care." Advocate for systemic changes that support postpartum women, such as paid parental leave, access to affordable childcare, and mental health services. Collaborating with policy-makers to push for maternal health equity helps dismantle barriers to proper care.
- **Promote Access to Culturally Competent Care:** Ensure that the care you and your colleagues provide is culturally competent and addresses the unique needs of women from different backgrounds. This includes being aware of traditional healing practices, cultural perspectives on motherhood, and promoting access to services that meet diverse needs.

4. Collaborate Across Disciplines for Integrated Care:

- **Interdisciplinary Collaboration:** Work closely with other perinatal professionals, including midwives, lactation consultants, doulas, mental health practitioners, and pediatricians, to create an integrated care network for mothers. By providing a united front of professionals who understand each other's roles, you ensure that mothers receive comprehensive care that addresses all aspects of postpartum health.
- **Shared Decision-Making:** Adopt shared decision-making models where the mother is at the center of her care, and each professional contributes their expertise while supporting the mother's autonomy. Encourage mothers to speak up about their needs, and ensure they feel supported by a team rather than burdened with the task of self-care.

5. Educate and Raise Awareness on the True Meaning of Self-Care:

- **Shift the Narrative:** Educate both clients and fellow professionals about the decolonized meaning of self-care. Instead of promoting the commercialized version of self-care (focused on products), emphasize the importance of rest, mental health, shared caregiving responsibilities, and community involvement.
- **Support Mental Health in Practical Ways:** Create awareness that real self-care includes mental health support, adequate rest, and help with daily tasks. Normalize asking for help, and create an environment where women feel comfortable reaching out when they are struggling.

6. Engage Partners and Families in Care:

- **Normalize Involvement of Partners and Family:** Help normalize the idea that postpartum care isn't just the responsibility of the mother. Encourage the involvement of partners, family members, and close friends in practical ways — from caring for the baby to supporting the mother emotionally. By making this collective support the norm, you can help reduce the isolation that many postpartum women feel.
- **Provide Education for Partners:** Offer education to partners and family members on how to support a new mother. This can include practical advice on household tasks, recognizing signs of postpartum depression, and how to provide emotional support.

7. Promote Sustainable and Accessible Self-Care Practices

Simple, Accessible Practices: Encourage sustainable and accessible forms of self-care that are less about consumerism and more about small, manageable steps like getting enough rest, going for walks, taking naps, or having a support system in place to help with childcare.
 Focus on Practical Needs: Instead of focusing on luxury self-care, support mothers in finding simple, realistic ways to care for themselves, such as taking short breaks when possible or relying on loved ones for help. Encourage family members to step in and provide tangible support like meal preparation or house cleaning.

8. Foster a Culture of Mutual Aid

Encourage Mutual Aid Networks: Foster the idea of mutual aid among clients, where mothers support one another with child care, meal sharing, or emotional support. Community-based mutual aid systems allow mothers to both give and receive care, helping to build a resilient, self-sustaining village around them.
 Professional Collaboration in Action: Actively collaborate with other professionals in your network to provide wraparound care for mothers. This means not only referring clients to other providers but also working together to design care plans that consider a mother's physical, mental, and social needs.

9. Respect Traditional and Cultural Practices of Care

Honor Traditional Postpartum Practices: Recognize and respect traditional forms of postpartum care, many of which focus on rest and communal care in the weeks after birth. Promote practices that honor the mother's cultural background and offer her the type of care that aligns with her values and traditions.
 Provide a Safe Space for Expression: Create a space where mothers from different cultures feel safe to express their needs and share their experiences without feeling judged or pressured to conform to mainstream ideas of self-care.

Nicole Longmire IBCLC PMH-C
@likeamotheribclc
www.mothernurturelactationservices.com

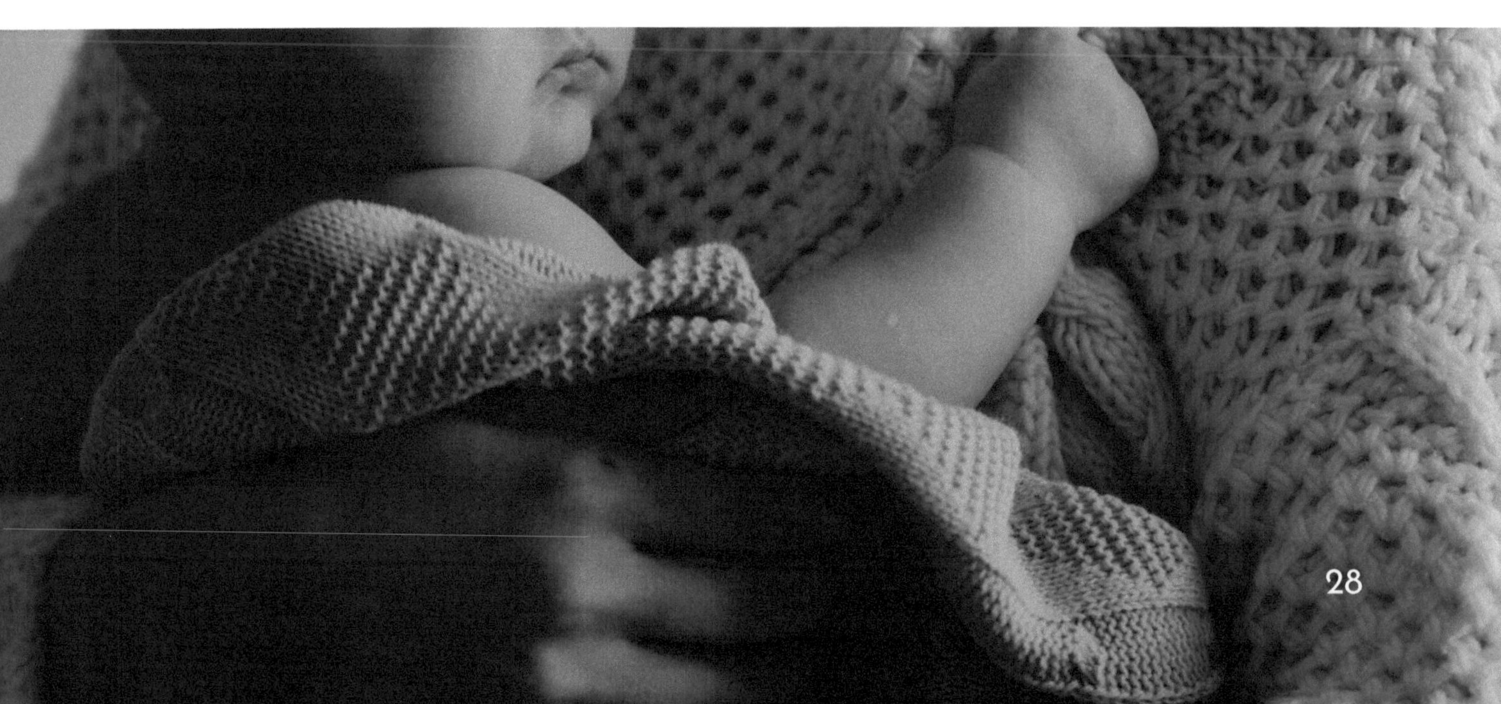

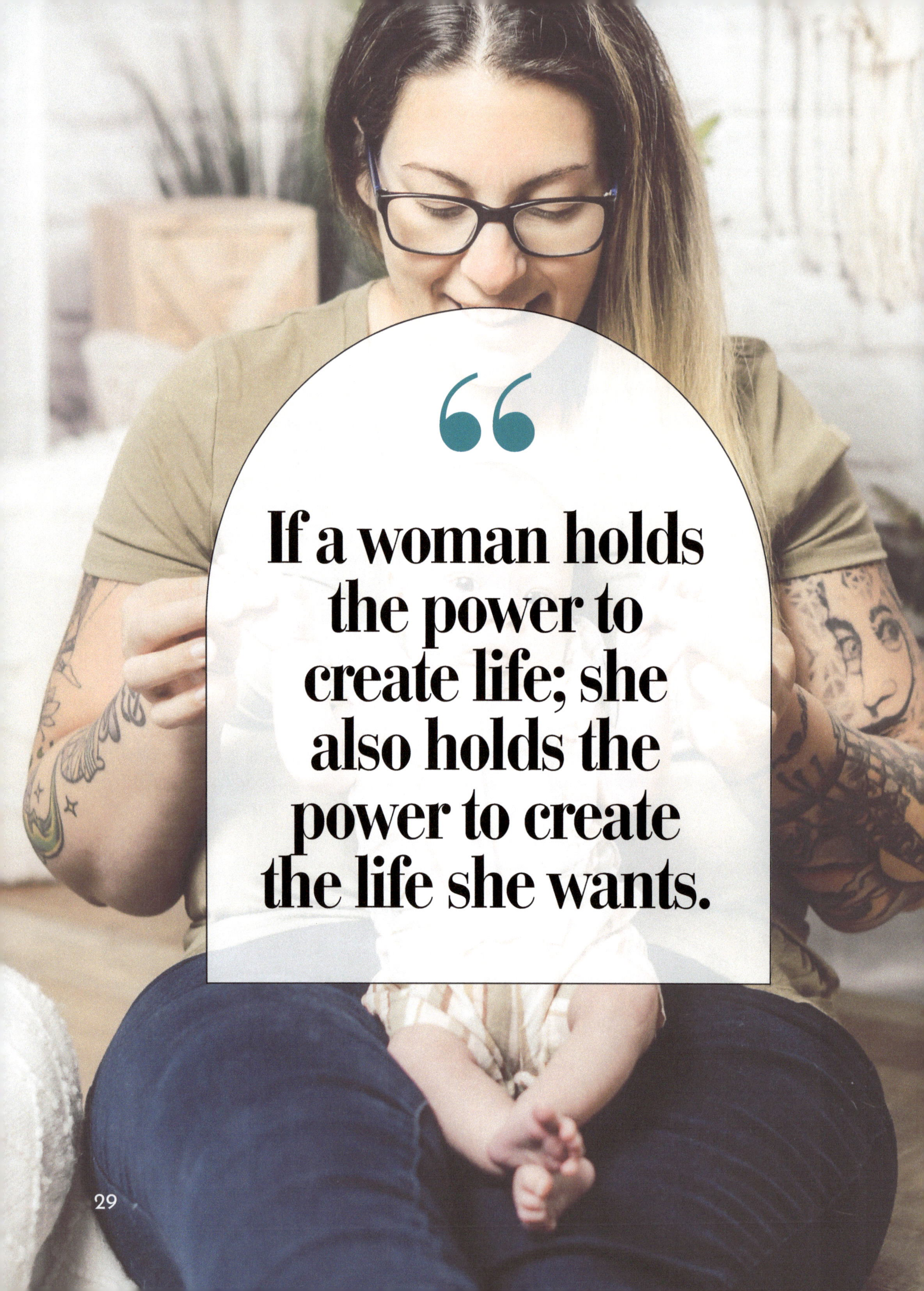

If a woman holds the power to create life; she also holds the power to create the life she wants.

The Ultimate Postpartum Healing Guide

Join us today and start your journey towards a stronger, healthier, and happier you!

By Rachael Van Schoick

Becoming a mom is a life-changing experience, and your postpartum recovery journey is just as vital as the pregnancy and birth itself. I get it—whether you had a C-section, vaginal delivery, or experienced perineal tearing, your body has been through a lot. At Align Movement, I'm here to support you every step of the way with exercises that are safe, effective, and tailored to your unique needs.

Understanding Your Postpartum Body

Before jumping into exercises, it's important to appreciate how much your body has changed. Each birth experience is different, and so is every recovery. Here's a quick rundown:

- **C-Section:** There are 7 different layers that were cut into during this surgery, so your recovery will focus on allowing those incisions and deeper tissues to heal. Which include scar massage, diaphragmatic breathing and gentle core activation at first. If this was an emergency C-Section don't disregard any feelings you may have about your experience, your mental health plays a vital role in how our bodies heal.
- **Vaginal Delivery:** If you had a vaginal birth, you might be dealing with perineal tearing or an episiotomy, or maybe even use of instruments to get baby out. Stitches will need care, attention and rest. Maybe you didn't experience any of these but are still dealing with a lot of swelling. Regardless of any situation, take into consideration your mental state as well, our bodies and minds play a huge role on how we heal.

First Steps: Gentle Movements and Self-Care

Rest, Hydration and Nutrition:
- **Rest:** Your body needs time to heal. Find moments to rest even if it's for a short amount of time. (I know easier said than done but set a timer if you have to and don't be afraid to ask for the alone time!)
- **Hydration:** Water is your best friend right now—which will help your tissue heal faster and help with milk supply if you are breastfeeding (you may not want to keep getting up to go to the bathroom, but this is extremely beneficial for your body, bowels and pelvic floor!)
- **Nutrition:** Nourishing your body every 2-hours is extremely important for tissue recovery, energy levels and milk supply if you are breastfeeding. (Feeding your body with protein, fiber, carbs and an arrayment of fruits and veggies can go a long way!)

Mental State:
No matter which method you gave birth to your new little one don't disregard your mental state. This can be about how your birth experience went vs what you expected, body image after baby, about baby and how you feel overall. Our bodies are so intelligent that they can feel when even the slightest mental shift isn't quite right. Don't be afraid to seek help and our bodies and minds will thank us for it in the end. Then healing can truly begin from the inside out.

Breathing Exercises: (This can start as early as day one if you are comfortable!)
- **Diaphragmatic Breathing:** This is your starting point for reconnecting with your core and relaxing your body. Lie on your back, knees bent, one hand on your chest and the other on your belly. Take deep, slow breaths, letting your abdomen rise and fall without your chest. Then focus on letting your chest rise and fall without your belly hand moving.

Pelvic Floor Exercises:
- **Pelvic Floor Connection:** Childbirth does have the ability to weaken your pelvic floor, but starting with gentle pelvic floor connections can help you regain strength if it's needed. Understanding how to do a pelvic floor contraction is where you start. The key to a pelvic floor contraction is that it needs to be just the pelvic floor contracting and nothing else. Remember this is just a starting point and only one way to assess. If any of these feel challenging at all it's time to get assessed by a professional like myself or a pelvic floor pt. There are various reasons to why we may or may not feel a contraction and some of us might need more contractability than others. Understanding what exactly your pelvic floor needs is extremely important to pelvic health.

Walking:
- **Short Walks:** Take short, gentle walks. It's great for circulation and helps prevent blood clots, especially after a C-section. Start with a short amount of time between 10-20 minutes, listen to your body and increase as you "feel" like you can. (If there is any increase in bleeding or discharge be sure to lessen the activity for that day and for the following, it's your bodies way of saying you did too much – reach out to your doctor if there is any pain or discomfort)

Gradually Reintroduce Postpartum Exercises
Once you're feeling up for it and have your healthcare provider's okay, you can slowly start adding more structured exercises. You could have the potential to start earlier then you might have been led to think.

1. Core Activation
2. Strengthening Exercises
3. Stretching and Flexibility
4. Posture & Alignment

Lymphatic Drainage
The best treatment/massage you can get after a baby is lymphatic drainage. Lymphatic drainage is crucial postpartum because it supports the body's natural healing process by promoting fluid balance, reducing swelling, and enhancing overall recovery. First, it helps to eliminate excess fluids that accumulate during pregnancy and childbirth, which aligns with osteopathic principles of maintaining proper fluid circulation for optimal health.

Second, lymphatic drainage aids in detoxification, removing waste and toxins from the body, which is essential for restoring balance and homeostasis. Lastly, it supports the immune system by encouraging the flow of lymph, which contains white blood cells crucial for fighting infections—an important consideration as the body heals postpartum. These principles emphasize the body's inherent ability to heal when given the right conditions and support. Reach out to someone in your area like myself who is trained in lymphatic drainage that can expedite your healing process.

Tailor Exercises to Your Needs:
There are a no one-size fits all approaches here. But here are some tips on where you can start. If you've had a C-section, focusing on posture, body mechanics and avoiding lifting heavier things other than your baby until you've healed fully can be extremely beneficial (at least 6 weeks for healing-some individuals might need more time before doing anything too strenuous.)

For those with perineal tearing, breathing and prioritize healing of your stitches, using ice packs within the first 12-24hrs and slowly getting back into pelvic floor work and pressure management will benefit you greatly. For those of you who have neither tearing, or a c-section can focus on reducing swelling in the body, posture, breathing and re-engaging muscles again. Your body just did an AMAZING thing. Appreciate it, listen to it and move in the desired direction YOU want, it's not a race, it's your body and it is strong and powerful. Just like you Mama!

Integrating Osteopathic Principles and ELDOA:
As an ELDOA trainer and someone deeply rooted in osteopathic principles, I believe in working with your body's natural alignment and structure to promote healing. ELDOA exercises are specifically designed to create space in your joints and spine, helping you feel taller, lighter, and more balanced. Incorporating ELDOA into your postpartum recovery can help address pain, improve posture, and enhance overall well-being. Creating strength and lengthening that will forever change your world.

Seeking Professional Guidance:
Postpartum recovery can be overwhelming, but you don't have to do it alone. A postpartum specialist like myself can create a personalized plan that ensures you're doing exercises safely and effectively. With the right tools you can get back to anything you desire. Which can leave you feeling even better than you did before pregnancy!

Ready to Take Your Postpartum Recovery to the Next Level?

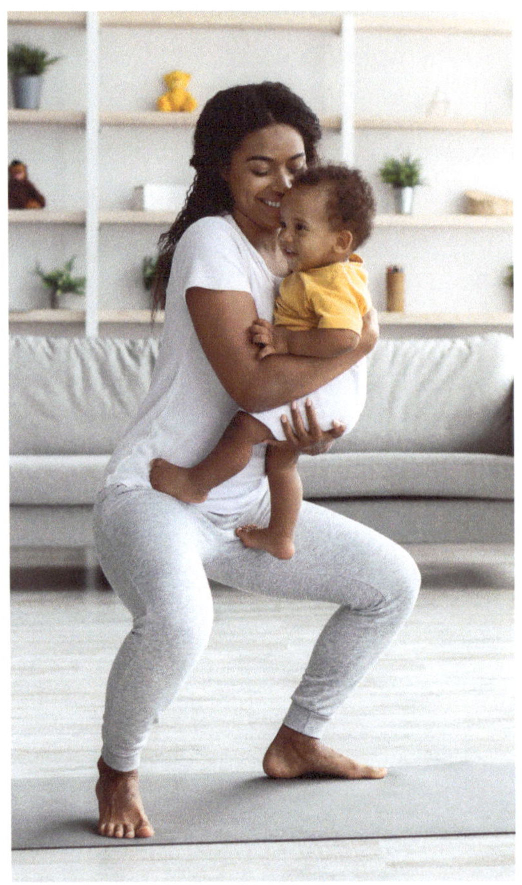

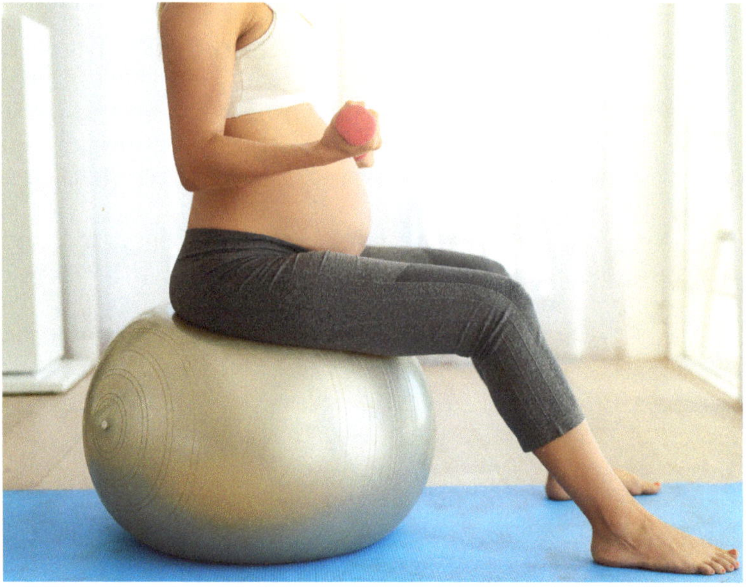

My "Power in Postpartum" program is here to help you regain strength, boost your confidence, and return to the activities you love. Over 8 weeks, we'll focus on exercises tailored to your needs, supported by professional guidance and a community of moms just like you. With a blend of core activation, strength work, ELDOA, and mindful movement, you'll heal faster, feel stronger, and be ready for anything.

Join us today and start your journey towards a stronger, healthier, and happier you!

Learn more about the Power in Postpartum program and sign up now!

https://www.alignmovement.com/power-in-post-partum-get-info/

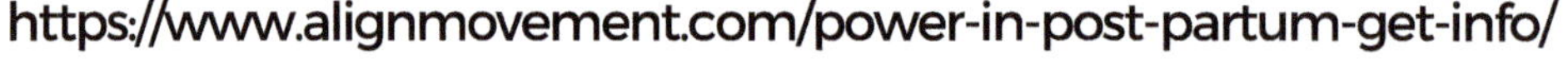

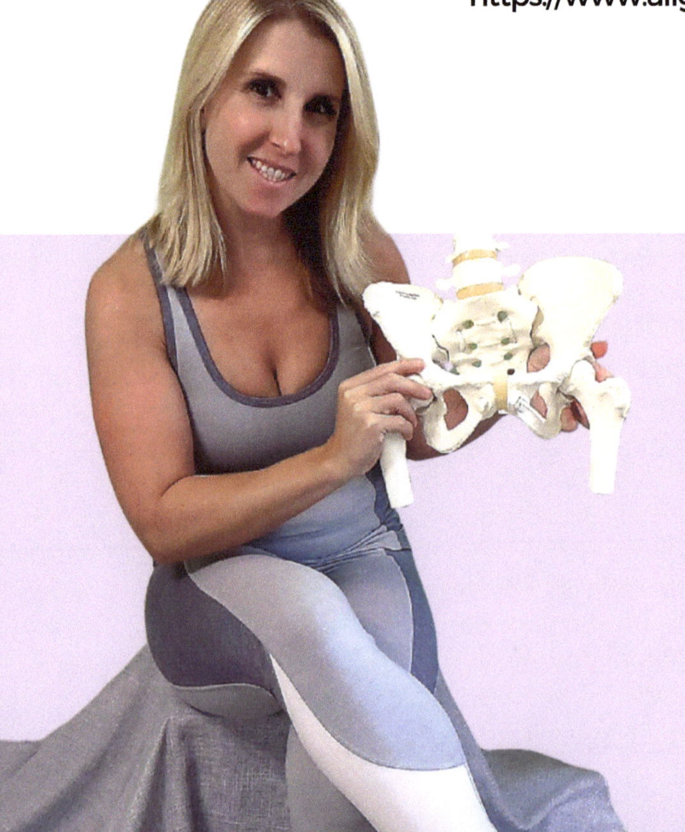

Rachael Van Schoick
Align Movement
LMT, Birth Doula, Prenatal and Postpartum Exercise Specialist, SomaTrainer and ELDOA Trainer

@alignmovement_therapy
https://www.alignmovement.com/

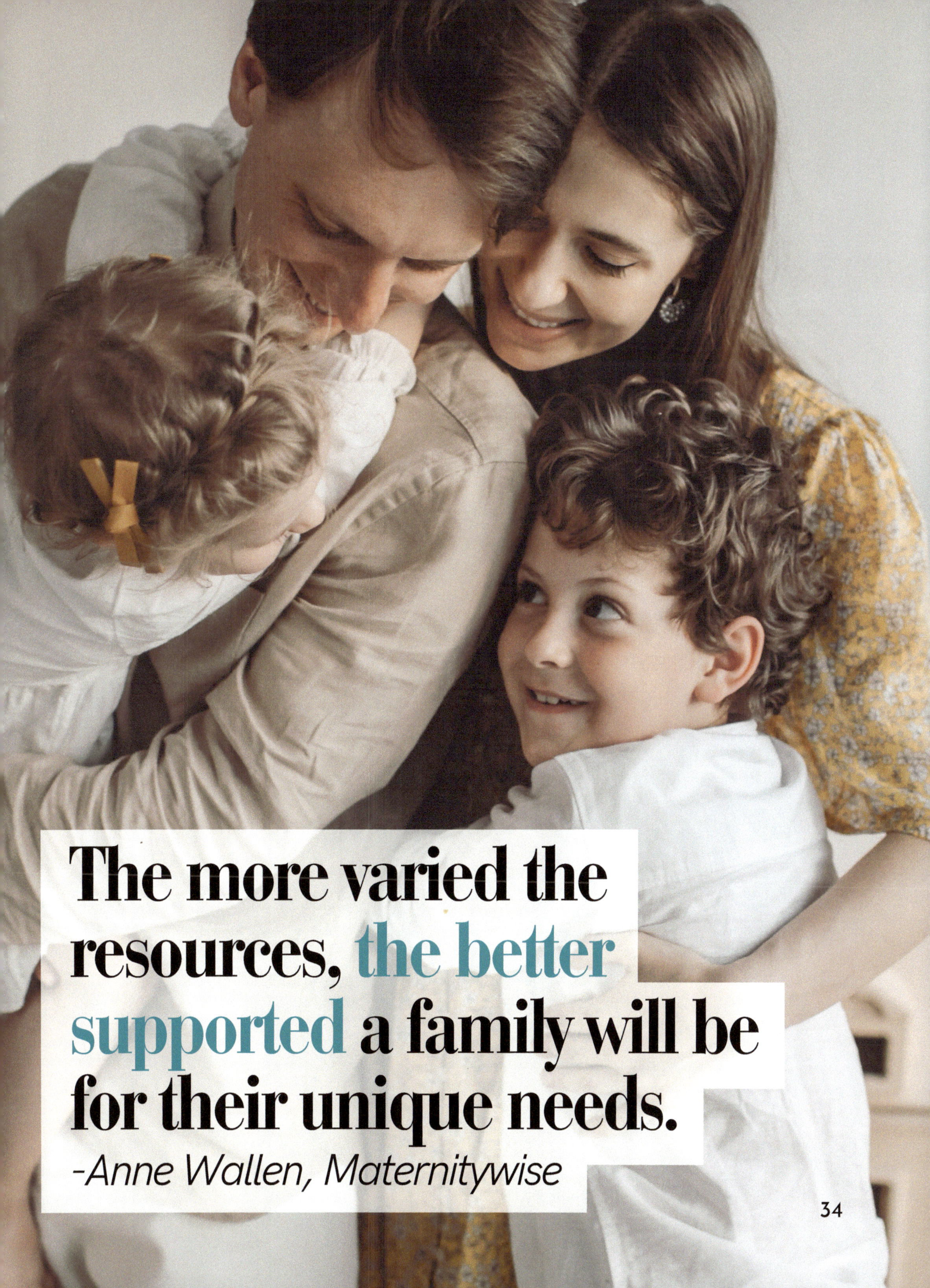

The more varied the resources, the better supported a family will be for their unique needs.
-Anne Wallen, Maternitywise

ADHD and the Womb-Centered Coach: A Journey of Chaos, Creativity, and Compassion.

By Kim M. Morris

Alright, let's talk ADHD—specifically, ADHD as a woman, a womb-centered coach, and a female entrepreneur. If you're like me, juggling a thousand thoughts a minute while trying to maintain some semblance of order in your life, you know this isn't for the faint of heart. But hey, if we're going to ride the ADHD rollercoaster, we might as well make it fun, right?

The ADHD Struggle is Real (And Sometimes Hilarious)
Let's be real: ADHD isn't just about getting distracted by shiny objects or losing your keys for the millionth time (though, let's be honest, that happens). It's about trying to focus on your next big project while your brain is playing a game of "let's think about everything else instead." It's starting a task with the best intentions, only to find yourself an hour later deep in a YouTube rabbit hole, learning about how wombat poop is cube-shaped (yes, it really is). As a womb-centered coach, you're probably tuned into your body and emotions—but ADHD has a way of throwing a wrench into even the best-laid plans. One minute you're channeling your inner goddess, meditating on your divine feminine energy; the next, you're frantically trying to remember if you fed the cat or emailed that client back.

Coping Mechanisms (a.k.a. Surviving the Chaos): So how do we, the neuro-spicy women with ADHD, manage to stay on track? Here are some coping mechanisms I've picked up along the way, sprinkled with a dash of humor and a whole lot of understanding:

Embrace the List (But Keep It Short, Sweet, and Maybe Sparkly): Lists are your friends, but let's not get too ambitious. Start with three main tasks a day. And if you're feeling fancy, add some stickers or colors—anything to make it fun. Trust me, crossing things off feels like winning at life.

Timers Are Your BFFs: Set a timer for everything. Seriously. Whether it's 15 minutes to focus on work or 5 minutes to actually find those keys, timers help keep you anchored in reality (instead of floating off into the land of endless possibilities).
- **The Pomodoro Technique (Or as I Like to Call It, the "Tomato Timer Thingy"):** Work for 25 minutes, take a 5-minute break, repeat. It's like tricking your brain into thinking it's a game, and who doesn't love a good game? Plus, those breaks give you a chance to dance it out or have a mini-snack fest.

Outsource Your Memory (No, Really): Apps, planners, sticky notes—use whatever you need to remember important things. I've got reminders on my phone for everything, from "send that invoice" to "take a breath." Because let's face it, sometimes even breathing feels like something we might forget.

Celebrate the Little Wins: Did you finally send that email? High five yourself. Remembered to drink water today? You're basically a hydration queen. Celebrate every little win, because with ADHD, it's all about the small victories.

Be Kind to Yourself: ADHD is a part of who you are, and that's okay. Some days will be harder than others, and that's okay too. Remember, you're doing your best, and that's enough.

ADHD Superpowers: Yes, You Have Them! Now, let's flip the script. ADHD isn't just about struggles; it's also about strengths. Here's where you get to embrace your superpowers:

- **Creativity On Steroids:** Your brain is a powerhouse of ideas. Sure, they might come all at once in a chaotic mess, but that's where the magic happens. You can see connections others might miss, and that's a gift.
- **Hyperfocus (When It Kicks In):** Ever get so engrossed in something that you forget to eat? That's hyperfocus, baby! Use it to your advantage—just maybe set a reminder to come up for air once in a while.
- **Empathy and Intuition:** Living with ADHD gives you a unique understanding of other people's struggles. As a womb-centered coach, this empathy is pure gold. You can connect with your clients on a deeper level, offering them the support they need.

Wrapping It Up (Before We Get Distracted Again): So, there you have it—a mix of chaos, creativity, and compassion. Being a woman with ADHD, a womb-centered coach, and a female entrepreneur is a wild ride, but it's one we're uniquely equipped to handle. Remember, it's okay to laugh at the struggles, celebrate the successes, and most importantly, be gentle with yourself along the way. After all, if we can juggle all of this, we can do just about anything. And if we forget a thing or two along the way? Well, that's just part of the journey. Here's to thriving in our beautifully messy, ADHD-infused lives!

Kim M. Morris

Yoniversity Online Training Academy
Womb Centered Coach, CEO

@yoniversityonlineacademy
www.yoniversity.us

> " **It's okay to laugh at the struggles, celebrate the successes, and most importantly, be gentle with yourself along the way.** "

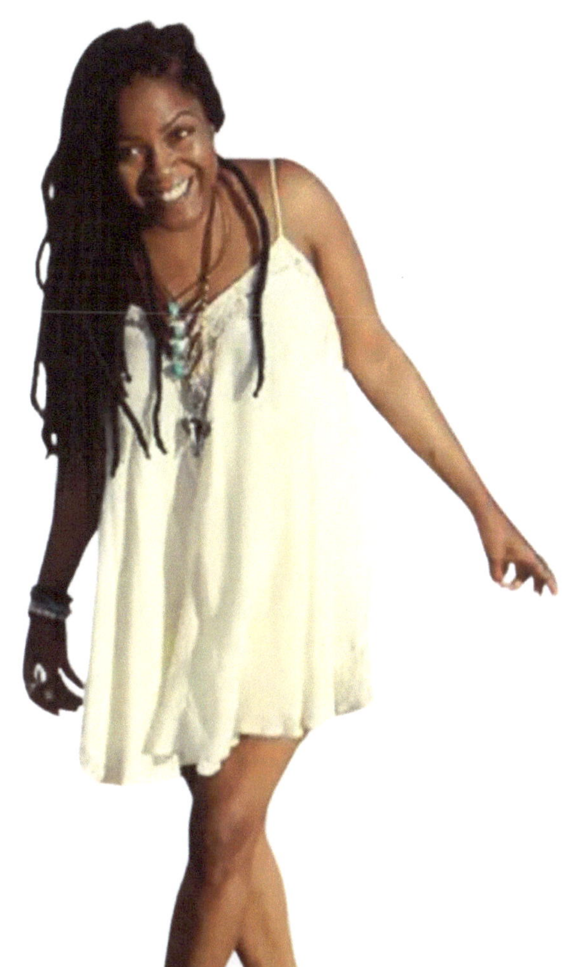

It Truly Does Require a Village

By Lisa van der Wilt

Truly, I tell you, it takes a village to raise a child. This saying has been tossed around for quite a while now, and even though I've been working as a doula for only five years, I believe it so much more now than I ever did at the start. I wanted to share a story that resonates quite close to my heart, and it's from my early days working as a doula. Actually, it's a story about the very first family I helped as a postpartum doula.

Now to take you back, this was some time ago. I was only 18. I had decided that I was going to quit university, leave the world of business behind, and then lo and behold, I actually decided to do the opposite and start my own. When I heard about doula work, I didn't really think it was a job. I believed it was more like a childbirth educator or babysitting... but when I took my course with Bebo Mia, I learned that I was wrong.

I created my website, started a social media presence, and after only a couple of months, I received an inquiry. This was from a couple in their late thirties who wanted to have a postpartum doula. Her family was not very close with her, and she knew she wanted extra support and help since she hadn't been around children much in her life. I can't begin to tell you how nervous I was. Only two years before that, I believed every time I held a baby, I was going to drop it. (Isn't this always the case?) After my initial consultation with them, we connected really well, and they knew they wanted to hire me. I had been honest that my skill level was not that of others they may interview, but they didn't care as long as I knew what I was doing and had worked with babies before. (I had been a babysitter since I was 13, so I felt I had it in the bag.)

Regardless, their baby was due in a month, so I had some time to prepare myself and review my classes once more. Some time passed, and when I got the call to tell me my first shift was starting a couple of days later, I was thrilled. It turned out the baby came early and had been born the previous day. Being as excited as I was, I barely slept that night! When I left for their house that morning, I was confident (or, well, I was going to fake it until I made it!)

Once I stepped through the door, it felt chaotic. They were overtired, and you could sense it. I asked how they were doing and what they needed in that moment. It turned out that since the baby came early, they wanted my help building the playpen. Now mind you, I had never built a playpen, but they seemed desperate and defeated if it didn't get done. So I metaphorically rolled up my sleeves and jumped in. Each shift afterward was filled with surprises. One time, the father pulled me aside and asked for guidance and information regarding the baby's eating patterns and whether the child was getting enough. He was so stressed about it, but with the little information I knew and shared, he calmed down, like the conversation was enough to put him at ease.

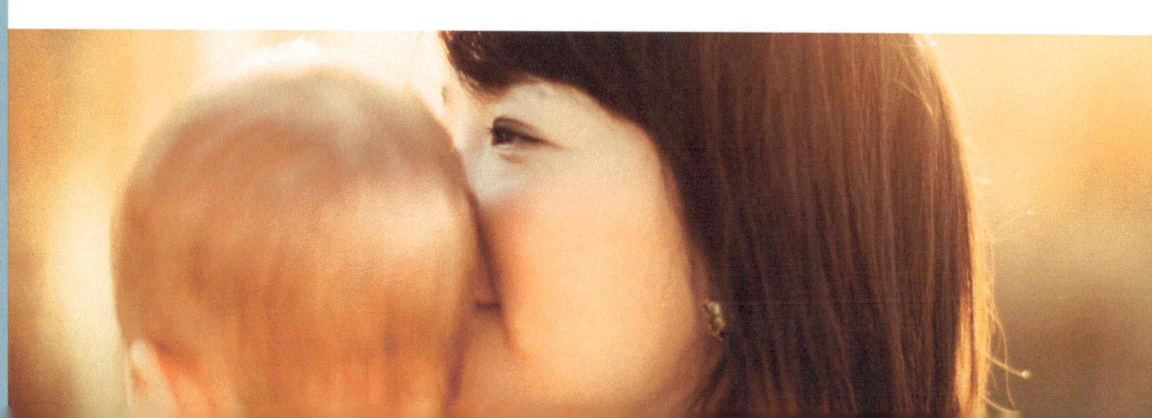

The amount of times they leaned on me so they could just take a shower in peace, have a nice home cooked meal - of course, the father was a chef, so this made me panic as I was no five star restaurant you know... actually I may have even used that line.

I also had the privilege of giving the baby's first bath with them present. He was so tiny and having only weighed a little over five pounds, it was such an experience. Then, on another visit we had an impromptu photoshoot. I hadn't any knowledge on professional photography but the fact that their photographer was busy and couldn't come early for them, I did what I could.

I learned so much from them and when the time to say goodbye came, it broke my heart. But it never really was goodbye. Her family lived close to mine and we passed the level of business to that, one of friendship.

She had communicated with text quite often sending updates about their family and how things were going. The kicker came when a couple of months later I received a phone call from her. Strangely, quite out of the blue.

It turns out they were going to be having a second child... it seems she was repeating a story similar to that of my mother who had my sister and I only sixteen months apart.

She mentioned how she would need my support once more, and I felt so glad to be doing it for them. Hell, this time I knew what I was doing. I wasn't nervous and I could actually be of some use to them or so I thought.

She had wanted my help before the child was born as more of a mother's helper inside the house, supporting the seven -or - eight month old (okay it's spotty I forget his age) with basic necessities.

Our plans changed some, originally I was planning to go to the hospital with them, older sibling and all my role would have been to take care of the child and be help for them during delivery. With the world and its problems, it changed, and four thirty in the morning I went to their house to stay home with the little guy. By that evening dad came and watched him, so I could relieve him the following morning.

I was doing that for a few days leading up to them bringing baby number two home. I felt so blessed to be a part of all those memories, and to be so much help during the beginning.

In the end, it was quite different supporting her for baby number two. She was experienced, she knew what she doing, and at the time I felt as if I was useless, but looking back I know that for her, she was more than happy to just have me be there *in-case* she needed me for something big.

Support comes in many shapes and forms, and it isn't just black and white. I haven't had one family be identical to the next. Each situation looks different, but it all circles around to the same thing. Having more people there to guide you.

Maybe you have a doula, maybe a really good extended family as long as someone is there to hold you. Not just the baby.

In the end, all that matters is that you aren't doing it alone.

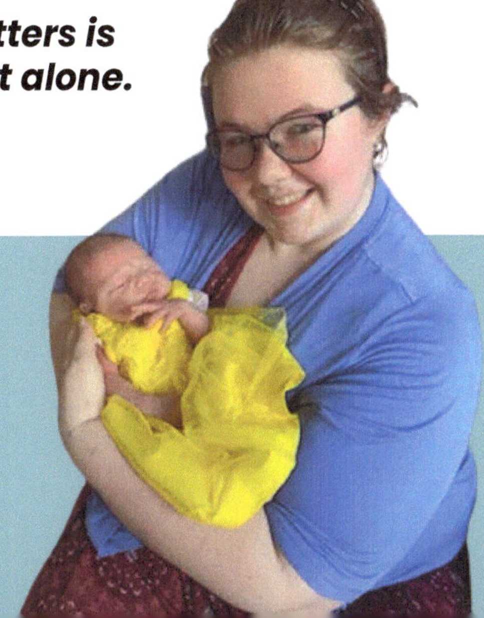

Lisa van der Wilt
Fruitful Womb Doula Services
Certified Birth, Postpartum, and Fertility Doula, Birthkeeper,
 Menopause Coach and Advocate, PLC
@fruitfulwombdoula
https://fruitfulwomb.ca/

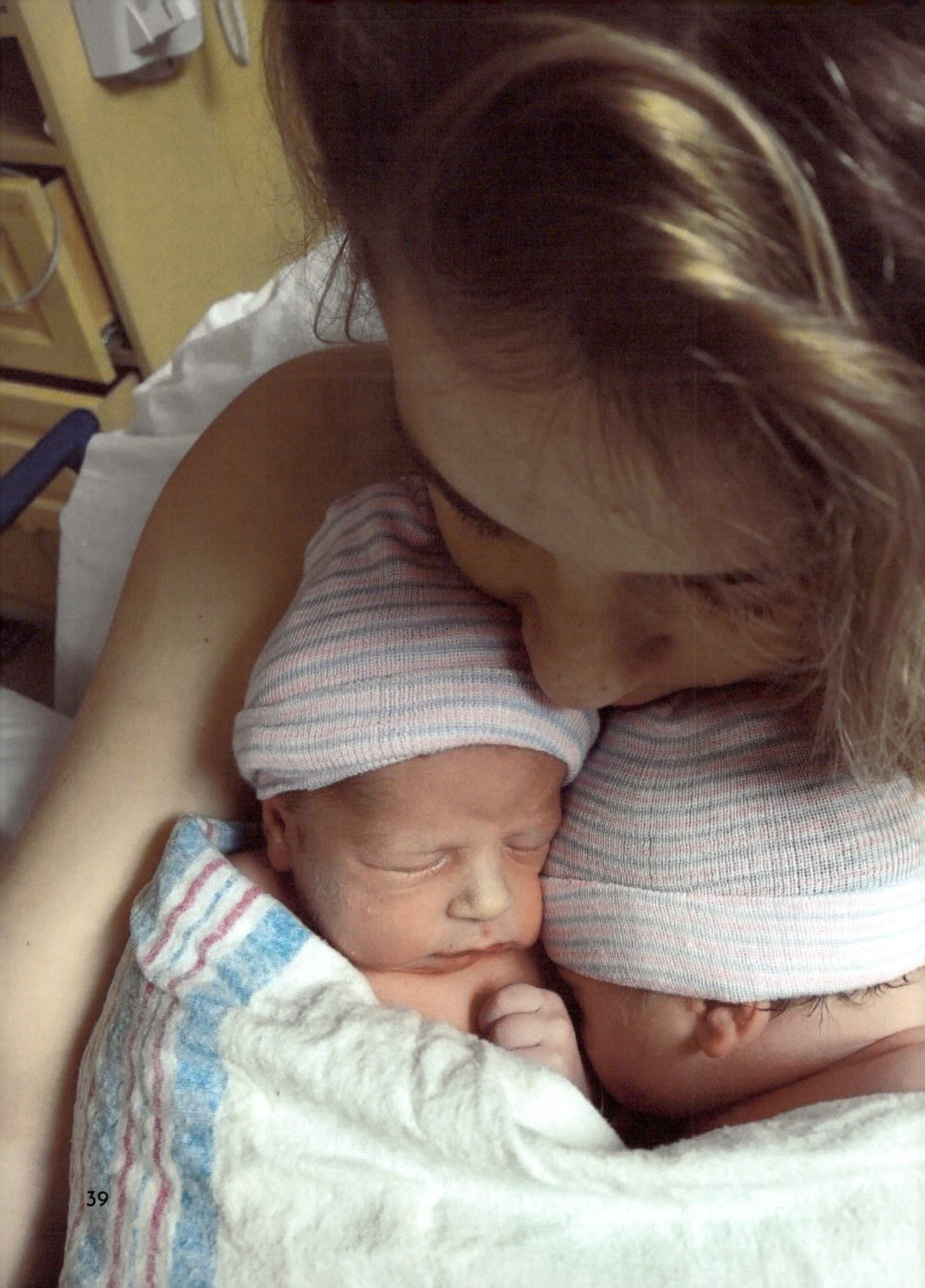

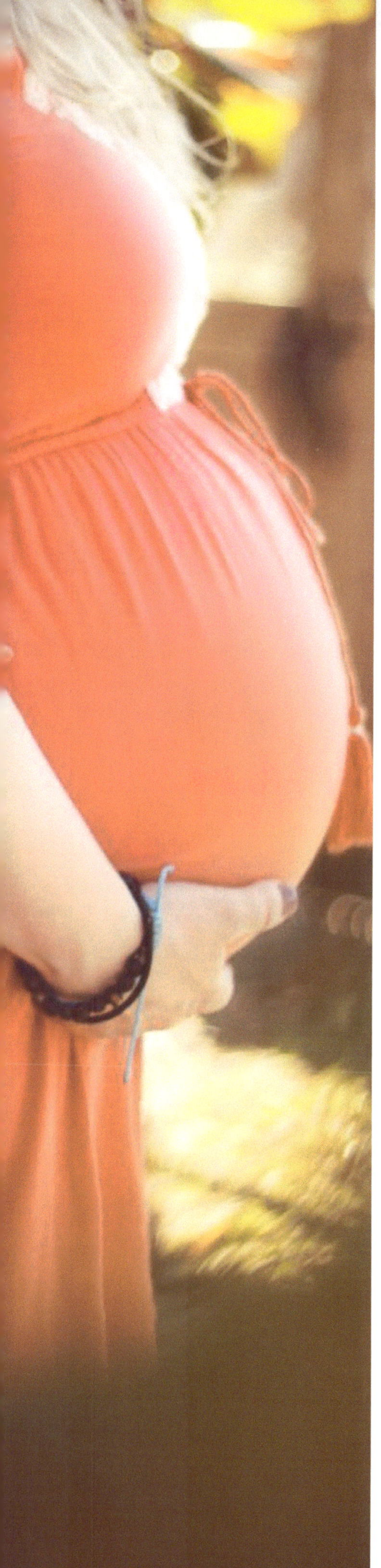

BEING PART OF A COMMUNITY

Everyone has their own reasons for becoming part of the birthing community. Whether your a doula, Midwife, physical therapist, or mental health facilitator. We all have one thing in common, **to build a community.**

A community where we are standing together for one purpose, to support mamas. I began my journey as a doula during the pandemic, it was hard, undeniably, it defeated my spirit because the policies had changed and work was not out there for me.

However, three years later I stuck with it finally received my certification. Then, I met a awesome group of women the Perinatal Resource Collective (PRC), and talk about support! These women are on fire with ideas, advice and willingness to help. We all are under the same understanding that we need to unite to make a difference. This is what I needed to start making a difference within my own community.

Being associated with PRC, has encouraged me not to only reach out to them for resources but my community as well. I am beginning, doula meet and greets, to spread the word of benefits of doulas in the perinatal community. I am reaching out to local resources to become, guest speakers, instructors, or offer their services to future clients.

Being a part of something can dramatically change your world 180° in the matter of weeks. If you are a new doula, one who is feeling down, or unable to see your fullest potential? Become part of this community of phenomenal women and just see how much you matter and how much you can make a difference within your community.

OUR COMMONALITY IS TO BUILD COMMUNITY

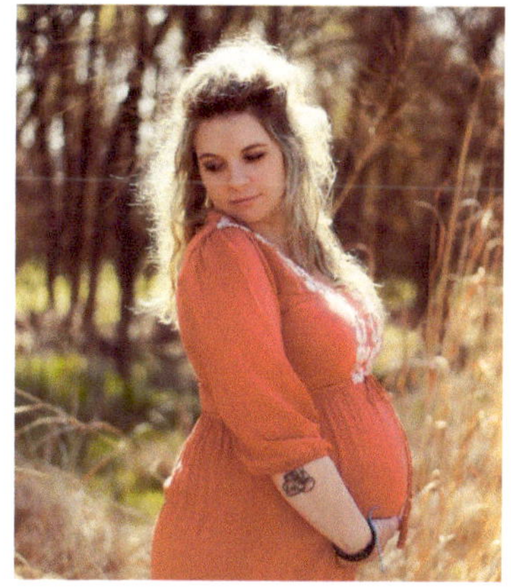

Sarah Kyle
Doula, CLD, CLSE
@confidentmamasdoula
confidentmamasdoula.com

40

building your village one episode at a time.
LISTEN NOW!
SPEAKING OF THE VILLAGE
PODCAST

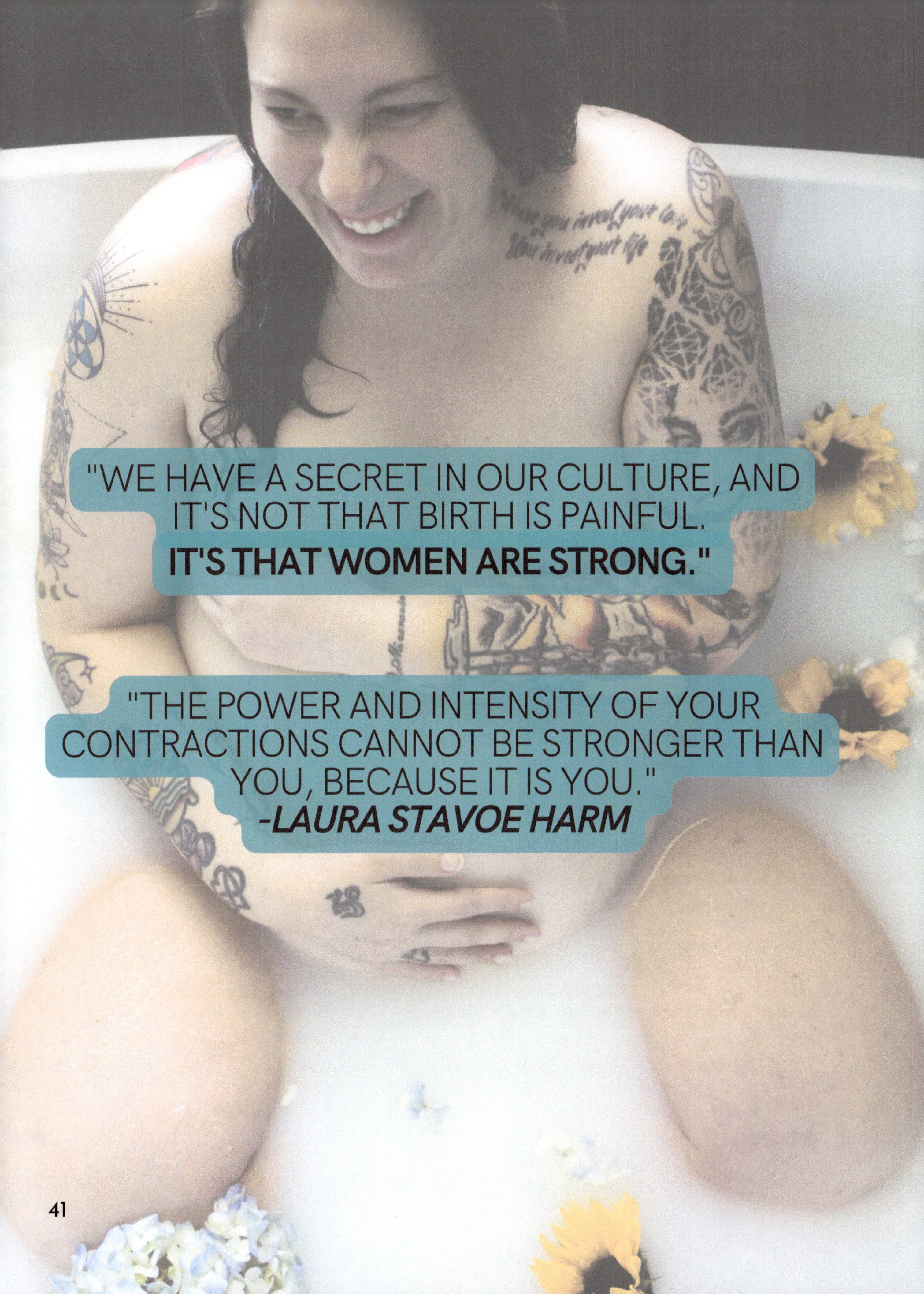

"WE HAVE A SECRET IN OUR CULTURE, AND IT'S NOT THAT BIRTH IS PAINFUL. IT'S THAT WOMEN ARE STRONG."

"THE POWER AND INTENSITY OF YOUR CONTRACTIONS CANNOT BE STRONGER THAN YOU, BECAUSE IT IS YOU."
-LAURA STAVOE HARM

THANK YOU!

From the bottom of my heart & womb, I am so grateful for every women, mother and supporter that is reading this magazine, has contributed to this magazine in some way, and for anyone sharing it!

The concept, implementation and distribution is not easy along with many other projects in the works but I am so excited for it to be live and for YOU to get even just one thing from these words.

I am hopeful that as the Perinatal Resource Collaborative grows and expands we will be able to offer issues more frequently but for now as the seasons are upon up, we will birth and deliver a new collection of resources, stories, and articles to share.

This is such a labor of love and a passion of mine- and I am thrilled to bring it to life.

Please provide any feedback and share with others if it has helped you in anyway!

If you are reading the print version of this in an office or place of business- be sure to scan the code below to subscribe to the digital version for free!

Nicole Harlet

xo